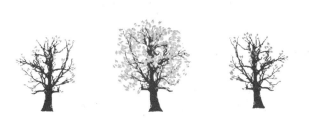

SHARED EXPERIENCES AND PRACTICAL ADVICE ON CARING FOR AGING PARENTS IN CANADA

Our Turn
to Parent

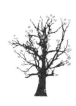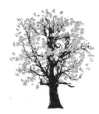

Barbara Dunn and Linda Scott

RANDOM HOUSE CANADA

www.randomhouse.ca

Random House Canada and colophon are trademarks

Library and Archives Canada Cataloguing in Publication

Dunn, Barbara, 1975–

    Our turn to parent : shared experiences and practical advice on caring for aging parents in Canada / Barbara Dunn, Linda Scott.
Includes index.

ISBN 978-0-307-35713-7

    1. Aging parents—Care. 2. Adult children of aging parents—Family relationships. I. Scott, Linda (Linda A.), 1961– II. Title.

HQ1063.6.D85 2009   306.874084'6   C2008-904126-7

Text design by Kelly Hill

Printed and bound in the United States of America

10 9 8 7 6 5 4 3 2 1

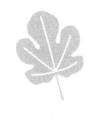

For our parents,
Bill & Eileen
and Dorene

CONTENTS

Introduction: Shared Experiences — *1*

1
Taking Care of the Generations — 7

2
Caregiving in the Early Stages of Aging — 25

3
Family Dynamics — 55

4
Helping Your Parents Stay in Their Home — 77

5
Helping Your Parents Move — 97

6
Medical Issues — *127*

7
Financial and Legal Issues — *157*

8
You as Caregiver — *183*

Conclusion: The Rewards of Caregiving — 203

Acknowledgments — 207
Senior and Caregiver Resource Guide — 209
Endnotes — 253
Index — 255

INTRODUCTION

SHARED EXPERIENCES

We—Barbara and Linda—worked in the same office and talked every day about the normal things one talks about with co-workers—career, family, friends. And then, one day in 2006, our relationship changed. Barbara's eighty-year-old father was diagnosed with early stage Alzheimer's disease and soon her family was embroiled in a world of doctors, social workers and care facilities, a world of overwhelming and often confusing information. Family members had to come together and make decisions about what was best for their father, but also for their mother. It was an emotional time for Barbara, and because of the camaraderie already established, she felt that she could share with Linda some of what was happening. When she did, Barbara found that Linda too had a story to share.

Linda's seventy-seven-year-old mother lived with her and her husband and was an active senior. Linda had begun to notice small signs that her mother was aging: a cold that became a serious infection (should I talk to her doctor?), a stove burner left on (but don't we all forget at one time or another?). When Barbara started talking about her experiences it was a wake-up call for Linda, who realized that she was missing important information about her mother's plans and possible needs for the future. Who had her mom selected to have power of attorney for personal care? Where was her mother's will? What resources were available in the event that her mother needed formal care?

Barbara had to contend with a large family within which there were conflicting ideas as to what should be done to help their parents. Meanwhile Linda's only brother lived far away, so she was concerned that the weight of responsibility would fall on her shoulders.

As the months came and went, and the crisis in Barbara's family gradually subsided, we continued to talk. We discussed our fears, both for our parents and for ourselves. How would we manage? What would we do? What *should* we do? What clues about her father's illness had Barbara and her siblings missed? What was Linda missing even now? In those exchanges we found much more than information. We found reassurance and kinship.

As we shared our stories, we also started to listen to others around us, and discovered that many people in our office, in our neighbourhoods, and among our friends had similar concerns and were taking on similar responsibilities for their aging parents. Initially we didn't use the term *caregiver* to describe ourselves; we didn't even know the term existed. We didn't know that we were part of the 2.1 million people,[1] many of us women, looking after our elderly parents, or that the Canadian government is conducting research about us, "the boomer generation" and "the sandwich generation," and the impact that we, as caregivers to our parents, have on our society and our economy.

As the two of us helped each other to find a sense of hope and understanding, we realized that many other people, people like you, needed to realize that they are not alone.

You are part of a growing community. Be assured that there are others who know what you are going through—that you're experiencing good days and bad, and that you are doing the best you can.

You have taken on the responsibilities of caregiving because your parents are family and you love them. While you probably share other aspects of your lives with friends and co-workers and occasionally even strangers, you might feel that to talk about your parents' health and personal affairs is an invasion of their privacy. You may feel a sense of guilt and uncertainty and isolation in your role as caregiver. But by sharing stories you will discover that you are not alone—that others are experiencing similar emotions: love, anger, frustration, sadness, desperation, loneliness.

Back in 2006 we found in each other someone who understood, someone who, although she was not going through exactly the same scenario, also had a story to share and an ear to lend. And even during the most frustrating or saddest times we had someone who could help us to see glimmers of humour. But what neither of us could find was a book to guide us through the decisions we were being called upon to make. We wanted a quick reference, a place to find specifically Canadian information to help us make those difficult decisions. We wanted a book of shared experiences and community.

So we decided to write it. *Our Turn to Parent* highlights the key areas that you, as a caregiver, need to be aware of and involved in during the early stages of your parents' senior years, and also discusses the situations and choices you may face as your parents move into their later senior years.

Everyone's experience is unique, and we are each at different stages of caregiving, yet what we share is that we are all trying to do what is best for our parents with the resources we have. We, the authors, are not experts. Like you, we are trying to find our way. What we've included in this book are the resources and information we wish we had had *before* we became caregivers to our aging parents. While it can't provide you with easy answers to the questions you will face, this book can provide suggestions and resources to help you through this life-altering journey.

Sadly Linda's journey as caregiver came to an end with the passing of her mom during the writing of *Our Turn to Parent*, but in these pages we both share our experiences. We have also collected the stories of other families from across the country. Our hope is in these personal stories you may hear an echo of your own situation, and find the kind of kinship that the authors discovered, and still share.

Where You Will Find Information

Most people do not have the skill sets and resources to act as care-givers on their own. If you're lucky enough to have professional caregivers, nurses or social workers in your family, be thankful, but more likely you will need to seek support systems. A tremendous amount of information is spread across many sources, including government agencies, community services, medical and finan-cial institutions, and the Internet. Often retrieving necessary and practical information is a confusing, time-consuming and over-whelming process. It's a great deal to sift through when you are in the middle of a crisis. We hope that in *Our Turn to Parent* you will discover a resource to reduce the confusion.

We explore the major caregiving issues that will confront you. Each chapter covers one of these issues and offers practi-cal information as well as tips, resources and personal stories that will allow you to further research your individual caregiving needs. Following an overview of caregivers and seniors in Canada, we explore how to

- be a caregiver to your parents in the early stages of aging
- work with your family to care for your parents
- help your parents stay in their home

- find appropriate accommodations for them when they can't stay in their home
- help your parents with their medical needs
- work with your parents to organize finances and legal documents
- look after yourself as caregiver
- appreciate the rewards of caregiving.

And at the end of the book we provide a Senior and Caregiver Resource Guide containing contact information for key national and provincial government and non-government organizations and services.

Our Turn to Parent is designed to supply you with information and resources you need as you care for your aging parents. Our hope is that our story, along with the stories of others across the country and even a few from around the world, will provide comfort and direction in the days ahead.

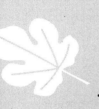

1

TAKING CARE OF THE GENERATIONS

No one can anticipate what it will be like for you the day you discover that you must become a caregiver for one or both of your parents. For Barbara, it happened the day her father experienced a sudden medical crisis. Although she had been aware that her parents were growing older, it wasn't until that moment that she realized she was going to have to be more intimately involved in how her parents lived their lives.

This is often how people stumble into the role of caregiver for their aging parents—suddenly and because of medical necessity. But others already are caregivers without even knowing it. Linda's mom was an independent senior, but Linda slowly came to realize that her small offers of assistance and regular telephone calls were the beginning stages of a more involved caregiving.

There are more than two million informal caregivers in Canada today ages forty-five and over.

If you've bought this book, it's likely you've also joined the community of caregivers. In this chapter we look at

- who caregivers are in Canada
- how the senior population is growing
- how seniors' lifestyles are changing

- how you parent your parent
- what your primary goals as a caregiver should be
- how you become a caregiver
- what the four stages of caring are.

Caregivers in Canada

One day you are busy with your life, pursuing your career, looking after your family, paying down your mortgage, and the next day your role changes and it's your turn to parent. If you are caring for a parent today, you are one of a growing number of Canadians who are looking after aging parents and who are defined by the government as "informal caregivers."

The role of caregiver affects all aspects of our lives: our work, our family, our time and potentially our psychological and physical health. It can be stressful and very emotional. It is estimated that informal caregivers save the Canadian public health system more than $5 billion a year by doing the equivalent work of 276,000 full-time employees.[3] Our work as caregivers also affects the companies we work for as time off work costs employers.

Family/informal caregiver is defined in Canada as an individual who provides care and/or support to a family member, friend or neighbour who has a physical or mental disability, is chronically ill or is frail.[2]

This official definition is limiting as it doesn't represent the different stages of caregiving.

The effect of informal caregiving is beginning to be addressed by our governments. For example, in 2008, caregivers were recognized in the Speeches from the Throne of both British Columbia and Ontario. New tools and support services were promised in B.C., and Ontario stated that it would provide a caregiver grant for those caring for elderly family members.

Women as Caregivers

The majority of caregivers in Canada today are women, though the number of men involved in caregiving is growing. In the past, women generally stayed at home to look after their family, and when parents became frail, the role of caregiver would be taken on by the daughters in the family. Now many women are working outside the home, yet still incorporating the role of caregiver into their lives in addition to fulfilling their responsibilities as mothers, wives and workers. This not only affects women as individuals but also has an impact on society on a larger scale. Businesses and governments need to start recognizing the growth in caregiving by providing more social programs and assistance so that the burden is not on the individual.

Approximately 70 percent of informal caregivers are women.[4]

The Growing Senior Population

A senior in Canada today is considered to be anyone aged sixty-five or over. Across the country we've eliminated compulsory retirement at age sixty-five because many seniors are still able to and want to participate in the paid workforce and are making a contribution to the economy and society. Also, many seniors still need to continue working because they are financially unable to retire.

Today seniors comprise 13.1 percent of the population.[5] Of this number, 1.5 million are seniors aged

Most people have their children raised before their parents need help, but my parents were much older by the time they had me. . . . What made it difficult was to be in my thirties with two small girls, two demanding jobs and looking after elderly parents at the same time. . . . However, if you have the means, the time and the will to care for your aging parents, do it. The reward is satisfaction.

JANET, NANAIMO,
BRITISH COLUMBIA

There are certain moments in my life that stand out as being significant: my first day of kindergarten, my high school graduation, and the day I moved into my first apartment. My mom, as the most important person in my life, was a part of each of those events. And she was there at the precise moment I officially grew up: the day she told me that she had stage-four breast cancer. That one conversation turned our world on its head—our traditional roles as kid and mom soon lost their meaning.

Over the years, while caring for and being with her, I had the privilege of adding to my collection of memories: the first time she allowed me to push her in a wheelchair around our neighbourhood block; the day she shared her signature chiffon cake baking secrets (it was on a Mother's Day); the first Thanksgiving when she sat back and declared me in charge of dinner festivities.

During this same time, we also had our share of lasts—some significant, but none nearly as important as those firsts. And as expected, our respective roles as parent and child swapped fully in due course. This inevitability was somehow inconceivable, yet befitting. Had we not taken this journey together, my list of firsts would be much shorter. And I wouldn't have officially grown up.

Some people may speak of duty or obligation when describing the role of caring for a parent. For me, it was a true honour to be in my mom's company. After all, she trusted me with this responsibility—me, her child! As an obstetrics nurse, wife and mother, she had looked after people all her life. She deserved only the very best care. How else could I better honour her? Only by trying to show the compassion and love that I learned from her perfect example.

SARAH, TORONTO, ONTARIO

When my mom turned eighty, we asked her to give up her licence. When she turned eighty-five, she had a heart attack and had to have a pacemaker put in, so my brother, sister and I take her where she wants to go. Now she is eighty-eight and I clean for her, she goes to the grocery store with my sister, and I take her to her doctor appointments. . . . Her grandchildren all help out as much as they can. My son cuts her grass for her. She doesn't want to go into a nursing home; she wants to stay at home.

NANCY, DRESDEN, ONTARIO

seventy-five to eighty-four, a number that has doubled since 1981.[6] These numbers are expected to grow. People are living longer today than ever before. In the 1900s the average lifespan was forty-seven years. Today our parents can expect to live well into their eighties.[7] Since people are also having fewer children, the senior population will be proportionally larger than in years past. It's no wonder everyone you to talk is either involved in or knows someone caring for an aging family member.

Seniors' Changing Lifestyles

The statistics show us that seniors are better educated, financially better off, and generally healthier than they were a quarter century ago.[8] Many of our parents have discovered the Internet and are using e-mail to stay connected to friends and family, as well as to access online information, and services such as those offered by retailers, that can make their lives easier.

How society views seniors is also changing. Many of the old stereotypes are being rendered obsolete. Seniors continue to work, and are healthy and active longer than in the past. Advertisements selling life insurance, medicine, cars and travel adventures portray seniors in active pursuits such as bike riding along a lake or mountain climbing.

Unfortunately it's easy for the rest of us to get caught up in the media image of the active senior and forget that we need to pay attention as our parents enter their early senior years. Every child, no matter how old, still tends to believe their parents are invincible. While we all hope that our parents will continue to be healthy and independent for a long time, we cannot ignore that they will eventually need our help.

The Caregiver in the "Me" Generation

Most of us lead busy, overscheduled lives and are often disconnected from our parents. Over the last couple of decades, people have become more transient and families are spread across the country and even the globe. As adult children going about our lives, we may not have thought that someday we would be asked to take an active role in the lives of our parents. This changing role comes as a surprise not because we don't care, but because we didn't observe the subtle changes as our parents aged.

How Do You Parent Your Parents?

As your parents age, you will be faced with many difficult decisions, and if you have reached the critical stage where you must parent your parent, then you are about to face one of the greatest challenges of your life. Your parents will come to rely on you more than ever as decisions need to be made, and you will move forward into a more active form of caregiving.

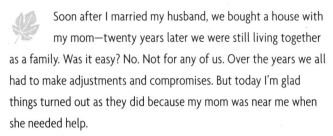

Soon after I married my husband, we bought a house with my mom—twenty years later we were still living together as a family. Was it easy? No. Not for any of us. Over the years we all had to make adjustments and compromises. But today I'm glad things turned out as they did because my mom was near me when she needed help.

My husband is an unusual man to have agreed all those years ago to move in with his mother-in-law. When we moved in we didn't talk about how long it would be. I asked my husband on and off in the early years if we should sell the house and move out on our own, but his reply was always the same: he knew I'd be happiest with my mom close to me, and besides, living together would be the only way he'd ever see me for all the visiting I'd do.

When I told people about how long we lived together, everyone marvelled at how we managed. How, they wondered, did my mom put up with my husband, or my husband with my mom, and how did I handle both of them? I've come to realize that they managed it for me, because they loved me. And as my mom got older and started to have some health problems, I thought, things happen for a reason. I'm so grateful to my husband who all those years ago said you'll be happiest if she lives with us.

LINDA

Your parents need to be involved in decisions and they need to be treated with dignity and respect. When to get involved, how much you are needed and how independent your parents can be are all complex questions. By approaching these questions with empathy for your parents, you will be able to make better decisions with more confidence.

The fact that it's "your turn to parent" doesn't suggest that your mother or father suddenly has become a child. It's essential you don't think of this new relationship with your parent as a role reversal. Rather, you will try to embody the attributes of a good parent in order to communicate and work through all the questions and emotions of these evolving situations. If you assume that you are supposed to take charge of your parents' life, answering all their questions and solving their problems for them, then you are headed for heartache. You will end up feeling angry that your parents are not showering you with gratitude. You will feel frustrated that they refuse to listen to your advice. If your parents were willing to share their lives with you previously, at this point they may start to exclude you. It will take understanding and effort on your part to work through these changes with them. Try to remember that your parents are independent people who have been leading capable and productive lives. Show them that you respect this.

OUR TURN TO PARENT

When it's your turn to parent you will

- be a guardian of and champion for your parents
- provide care and guidance
- listen and try to understand their point of view
- offer advice (not lay down the law)
- recognize that you can't control everything
- provide love and support.

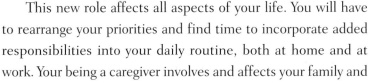

This new role affects all aspects of your life. You will have to rearrange your priorities and find time to incorporate added responsibilities into your daily routine, both at home and at work. Your being a caregiver involves and affects your family and

One day you are the child and then somehow, along the road, your parents become the children.

Sometimes it creeps up on you, like winter's long approach, and other times it happens overnight, like the ground giving out under your feet—ground that you never suspected wasn't solid. No one warns us this will happen, and even if they did, you still wouldn't be prepared.

Once it happens, the egg timer has been turned and you can't stop it. You try to make peace with all the unfinished business of your own childhood, you wonder how they got old so fast, and they look at you and think the same thing.

Some of us have children of our own and the new cycle brings us comfort. Watching all that youth spilling over into life reminds us of our own brief springtimes. Savour these moments because today they are kids, but before you know it, they may come to parent you.

CAREGIVER, TORONTO, ONTARIO

the many different relationships that exist within it. It will be a challenge trying to balance all these competing responsibilities and remember to care for yourself as well.

The Caregiver's Primary Goals

Two of the most fundamental factors in happiness are personal independence and dignity. Personal independence means being able to rely on your own capabilities, judgments and resources. It means that a person won't have the will of others imposed upon him or her. Personal dignity comes from self-respect and self-esteem. It means having confidence and a sense of self-worth. As a caregiver, your goal is to ensure your parents are able to maintain their personal independence and personal dignity. If these two ideals are the foundation for your behaviour, you will be able to keep focused and not get sidetracked by overwhelming decisions and emotions.

This does not mean that your parents will always be able to live on their own. You must consider their safety, and if that means that their living situation has to change, they (and you) may have to redefine what you mean by "independence." Even very frail or ill people can be encouraged to make small decisions to maintain their independence and dignity.

Taking an active role in making the decisions that have an impact on one's life gives one dignity. If your father needs meals delivered to ensure he is eating properly, then he should be part of the process of picking the meals and quantities and delivery options. Making these decisions cooperatively takes time and patience, but involving your parents in planning both big and small changes in their lives shows them that you have their interests at heart.

If you have ever been a medical patient, you will understand how quickly personal dignity can be lost. Maintaining your parents' personal dignity grows more difficult as their health deteriorates and you become increasingly involved in the intimate details of

When I am taking care of my father, it is as unpredictable as becoming a parent of a child. There are no books on the how-tos of this relationship, and you must learn as parents do—as you go. You just have your own ability to offer whatever you can to make their life happier. I became humbled when I saw the person I once knew become someone vulnerable and dependent. With this knowledge came trust and compassion. My dad was once a strong man and now needs my care. And you know what? I love it because he is more human and has developed all these interesting traits that I never saw before. Sure it's tough, and seniors may have their bad days, but as long as you don't take anything personally, they get over it and you just amuse them, and help them keep their dignity by not losing anything of themselves.

DEBORAH, CORNWALL, ONTARIO

their lives. But if we keep these priorities in mind, we can help our parents to maintain their personal dignity, honouring them and at the same time demonstrating to others how they should be respected.

As aging and ill-health erode your parents' abilities, concentrate on what they are able to do, rather than what they are no longer able to do. Look for ways to involve them in the tasks that you are doing for them. For example, if you have taken over paying the bills, perhaps your parents can open and sort the mail, reviewing the statements in advance. If you are doing the grocery shopping, take them along if they are well enough, and have them prepare the shopping list in advance. Unless they are medically incapacitated, or the situation is unsafe, there are always ways to work *with* your parents through all the aging stages.

THEIR GOALS ARE YOUR GOALS

Your aging parents want to

- maintain their personal independence
- maintain their personal dignity
- be seen by their caregiving children as adults, not as children
- focus on what they can still do, rather than on what they can no longer do.

Becoming an Active Caregiver

We each have a different level of involvement with our family, and these relationships change as we move through successive stages in our lives. Perhaps up to now you have interacted with your parents as an adult child with an independent life separate from them. You may attend family gatherings with your parents, participate in leisure activities with them, or help them periodically with jobs around their house—but in a way that fits into your lifestyle. At some point, though, they will begin to rely on you more, and your involvement in their lives will change.

Like us, you will eventually find yourself developing a different sort of relationship with your mother and father. The change may be subtle or dramatic. Perhaps your cooperative shopping trips become the only way they bring food into the house. Or maybe there has been a rapid decline in their health that requires you to become intimately involved with them in ways that at first feel uncomfortable for all of you. It won't always be obvious when you will need to step into the role of caregiver. As the years progress and your parents age, it is sometimes difficult to know whether changes you observe in your parents—absent-mindedness, a lingering cold—are natural or symptoms of a larger health issue. It's critical that you pay attention and watch for significant changes of any sort.

When and how should you step in? It's natural, at least at first, for you to feel helpless. There are so many interrelated issues that arise with respect to your parents' privacy, dignity and independence as you involve yourself in their personal lives, including their finances, medical care, lifestyle and even relationships. Your transition from adult child to caregiver for your parents will include many ups and downs. Few of us think ahead about this stage of our lives and theirs. You probably believed that you would always be the child in the relationship and that your parents

> The whole family felt very strongly about helping my husband's parents stay in their home as long as they could, and they both lived there until just prior to their deaths. On our days off, we often got groceries, had doctor visits, specialist appointments, and drove them where they needed to go. We all put our lives on hold to tend and care for Jack and Kay.
>
> JANET, NANAIMO,
> BRITISH COLUMBIA

would always be there to be relied on, to give you direction and to take care of you. You probably assumed that your parents would always be able to care for each other and that if they needed you they would ask. Life does not always turn out the way we expect or as we hope. We need to learn to adapt in order to do the best we can when facing these new challenges.

The Four Stages of Caregiving

As your parents age, you will encounter four stages of care, reflecting the aging process: time for planning, time for action, time for medical care, and time to say goodbye. Your new role of caregiver can start at any of these stages, and each will involve your time and effort, and you will find yourself needing to rearrange your life in small or large ways. Each requires you to provide a different level of care.

THE STAGES OF CARE

Time for Planning

YOUR PARENTS are independent but there are signs they need some assistance. They are in their early senior years, likely between the ages of sixty-five and seventy-four.

NOW IS THE TIME FOR having conversations with your parents about plans for their future. You are helping with chores around the house, running errands and looking for ways to make their home senior friendly.

AS A CAREGIVER you are starting to wonder whether the changes you see in your parents are normal for their age, and whether you should be concerned. You should start assessing their situation and helping them put plans in place for the future: preparing a will, evaluating their financial security, determining personal care wishes.

Time for Action

YOUR PARENTS are becoming less independent and rely more and more on you and the family for help. They are in their middle senior years, possibly between the ages of seventy-five and eighty-four.

NOW IS THE TIME FOR deciding whether they can continue to live on their own, and, if not, where they should live. Often in this stage you will be faced with a medical crisis and decisions will need to be made quickly.

AS A CAREGIVER you begin to identify yourself as a caregiver and to become more proactive. You will step in and start to help make decisions about your parents' situation. Your family, work and personal time will be affected. You will begin to deal with your parents' financial, medical and legal matters.

Time for Medical Care

YOUR PARENTS are in a medical crisis. This stage could occur at any age.

NOW IS THE TIME FOR interacting with doctors, specialists and family in order to make health-related decisions. You will also start making decisions with regard to your parents' care that could involve where they are going to live, what medical treatments are necessary and which life-sustaining procedures they wish to have.

AS A CAREGIVER you will find this to be the most difficult and time-consuming stage because of the complex nature of the medical and social services systems. Time off work, time away from family and stress may all be part of helping your parents during this stage. This stage may arrive slowly or dramatically, but it will be a highly emotional time for you and your family.

Whichever stage you are in, you'll find that it has its challenges. The first step is to recognize where you are and know what to expect.

All of these stages may happen, but not necessarily in the same way for everyone. Some people experience a medical crisis before they have recognized that their parents are showing signs of aging. They are then in the planning stage while concurrently dealing with a medical crisis. At some points you will have lots of time to make decisions but at other points you will have very little time. No matter which stage you're experiencing, there will be challenges, both practically and emotionally.

In the next chapter we discuss the early stages of becoming a caregiver.

> Every Saturday, I go to the local market with my mother. Fifteen years ago, my dad still came along until he had a stroke. Now that he needs a walker for support, moving around has become tougher for him.

Seeing them going through the aging process has been an interesting experience for me. Their routine hasn't changed, yet their steps have become narrower, their pace is slower and the lovely faces of my two darlings now have a tired aspect. Tired, albeit happy.

I know one day this routine will come to an end. But I hope that [day] doesn't come too soon, because this very routine is what makes me happy.

I feel guilty for not being able to keep them company more often. I try to be close to them, but my husband and kids also need me, so I am not with them as much as I wish.

My mom says: "Honey, go home to look after your affairs." And even when I leave, I know she is happy.

I realize that despite their chronological age they need affection and company. I don't want to see the clock ticking more and more, knowing that each minute going by means less time for us to be together. But I guess that's life.

I wonder if this happens to everybody?

SILVIA, SÃO PAULO, BRAZIL

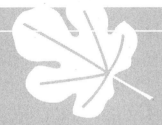

2

CAREGIVING IN THE EARLY STAGES OF AGING

Thischapter discusses how you will recognize when you need to step in as a caregiver. We look at

- encouraging good communication with your parents
- talking with your parents about their plans for the future
- becoming involved in your parents' decision-making
- paying attention to eating as an early sign that your parents need help
- driving as a hot-button issue
- recognizing the importance of social networks
- noticing signs that your parents need more help
- knowing when it is critical that you step in.

Communication in the Parent-Caregiver Relationship

How you communicate with your parents sets the tone for the way your relationship will progress as you deal with the issues of aging. Good communication will smooth the transitions and help you to put plans for the future in place.

The role of caregiver in your parents' lives is not an easy one, nor in most cases will it be short-term. You don't arrive one day and efficiently make all the decisions and then walk away. If only it were that simple! Before the role is suddenly yours, stop and think about the relationship you have with your parents and what you are willing to provide them emotionally and physically. Take an honest look at your relationship with them and the dynamics among your family members. Understanding the true nature of your relationship with your parents will help you to anticipate possible reactions and to recognize how to deal with the conversation. You also need to find out how your parents envision their future.

 Spend as much time together as possible. To get answers to all your questions, have awkward conversations. Once they are gone, any unanswered questions remain with *you*! Make peace, have no regrets and appreciate life for what it offers—good and otherwise!

SHEILA, GRIMSBY, ONTARIO

Having the Conversation about Aging

If you've never learned how to talk with your parents person to person, now is the time—and the conversation often begins with a frank talk about aging and what their wishes are for the future. Many adult children don't have this conversation early enough, either because they don't recognize that their parents need help, or because they are uncomfortable with the prospect of a discussion that represents a shift in the parent–child relationship. Acknowledging that your parents are getting older or need your help means acknowledging that your life is going to change too. It's scary to think that your parents may not be prepared for what the future holds and to know that you might one day be paying their living expenses or even making life and death decisions on their behalf.

But the experts, as well as those who've been through it with their parents, advise not to wait.

The truth is there is no perfect time—the right time is now. And it may in fact go better than you anticipate. You may

> Have the talk with your parents before the situation gets desperate and they are beyond making their own decisions. Make sure that all of the family is aware of their choices in order to avoid conflict before your parents become cognitively and/or physically impaired. Know where important papers are kept, what assets are involved, and your parents' wishes for their eventual distribution. And while you're at it, put your own life in order. It can never be too early for this, but it can certainly become too late.
>
> LESLIE, TORONTO, ONTARIO

be relatively surprised to find that your parents don't need as much help as you feared. They may have everything planned out and paid for so all you have to do is execute their wishes. But you won't know until you talk about it.

Talking now, even if the conversation starts out small, will benefit everyone later. The more you talk to your parents about getting older, what the future is going to bring, how they feel and what they've got planned, the easier it will become. You can slowly develop a new level of trust that as the years progress will become invaluable to you in helping your parents maintain an independent life.

Obstacles to Communication

Why, you may wonder, is everyone saying this conversation is going to be difficult? Surely your parents will understand that you are only trying to look out for their best interests and to take care of them? But remember that our generation was raised in a different time when people are accustomed to revealing intimate details on the Internet, through blogs or on websites such as Facebook. Most of our parents, on the other hand, were brought up to believe that what goes on in their lives should remain private. They may not want to burden their children with their health or financial issues, and as a result they may not reveal at the early stages how much help they may need.

Misunderstandings and hurt feelings will result if you don't respect your parents' values. Obstacles to mutual understanding can be both generational and cultural. You will need to understand and recognize them to have a successful conversation with your parents. You may face any number of scenarios.

If you are dealing with both your parents, you will likely encounter a strong reaction from your father, if he has been the provider and protector of the family, a role he will not be ready to relinquish to any of his children. It is not easy for men to admit that they are no longer capable of taking care of themselves or their families.

If your parents have not planned ahead, they may be embarrassed to reveal their circumstances to you. And if your mother is on her own, she may want to protect the memory of your father and not reveal that they didn't prepare for a future when he'd be gone. Be sensitive to this possibility and don't be judgmental if this turns out to be the case.

If a medical crisis has brought you to the point of having this discussion with your parents, don't be surprised to learn that health issues have been going on for some time and that your parents have kept them from you.

> It was not easy to live through seeing my father, who had always been very set in his traditional ways and used to helping his children, depending on his daughter for help. My father would not give up picking up the grandkids from school every day and even scheduled his appointments around the kids' schedule. He felt he could not miss it even if he was not feeling well. He would tell me it was his job and we could not take it away from him. We coped and took my dad's condition day by day. It was not easy on us but it did make us stronger as a family. Eventually my dad started to confide in me about what would happen when he was gone and how I would be taking care of my mom.
>
> MARIA, MISSISSAUGA, ONTARIO

Talking About Your Parents' Plans for the Future

Keeping in mind that the goal is to share a dialogue in which your parents feel safe and comfortable opening up to you, how are you going to approach them? The first step is to decide when to hold the conversation. Start by letting your parents know that you want to have an important discussion with them, and decide on a mutually convenient day when everyone has plenty of time set aside and there are no other conflicting appointments or stressful events taking place within the family.

If you feel you need to ease into the topic, share with your parents stories about friends and co-workers who have told you about the problems created when they were suddenly in a position to make decisions for their parents but didn't know what they truly wanted, or didn't have important information on hand

GOOD COMMUNICATION SKILLS

- Try to remain neutral. Strong emotions may get misinterpreted.
- Be honest.
- Don't manipulate information to make a bad situation sound good, or a good situation sound bad.
- Listen actively. Repeat back what's been said, ask questions and request feedback.
- Simplify language if necessary to ensure messages are clear, without being condescending.
- Offer advice, not ultimatums. Assist in researching solutions.
- Use positive body language: maintain eye contact, show concern in your facial expression.
- Use physical contact to give support.

at times when decisions needed to be made quickly. Let them know you don't want to be put in that position. Assure your parents that you are there for them and that you want to work with them to safeguard their independence and see that their wishes are carried out.

If the conversation doesn't go well the first time, don't give up: try again. If you believe your parents' situation is unsafe, or that action needs to be taken immediately, seek outside help from other members of the family, your parents' doctor, or your local social services agency (see our Senior and Caregiver Resource Guide under your province for listings).

Who in the Family Is Having the Conversation?

If you have siblings, contact them before initiating this conversation to share with them what you plan to do and why. You may find that someone else in the family is better suited to approaching your parents about this difficult subject. You and your siblings should meet and agree on what goals you hope to achieve and how to proceed. Consensus needs to be reached before you talk to your parents so that the conversation isn't sidetracked by bickering and other family issues. We talk further about family dynamics in Chapter 3.

Getting Help with the Conversation

If you have a dysfunctional family dynamic it's best to admit that up front and not try to take on this complicated and emotional discussion. If you believe that neither you nor another member of the extended family will be able to conduct this conversation, there is nothing wrong with seeking outside help from the outset. Talk to the family lawyer or doctor, or contact a family counsellor, any of whom will be familiar with these sorts of situations and can either advise you on how to proceed or even lead the discussion. It's important that you admit to the reality of your family relationships.

What the Conversation Is About

When you are ready to sit down with your parents, the first priority is to discuss what they have in place for their future. This includes their

- legal arrangements
- finances
- living arrangements and personal care
- end-of-life wishes.

Make sure your parents are aware that you are concerned about them, that you are not trying to take control of their lives but want to help them maintain the life they have for as long as possible—and to see their wishes fulfilled when the time comes and they are not able to advocate for themselves.

LEGAL ARRANGEMENTS

In order to take on this caregiving role you need specific information. You should determine whether your parents possess the following: a will, a power of attorney for personal care, and a power of attorney for property. If your parents do not have any one of these prepared, contact a lawyer as soon as possible. If your parents have prepared these documents, you should find out where they are kept in the event you need to access them, especially the power of attorney for personal care because it identifies who will speak for your parents during a medical crisis and they are unable to speak for themselves. Your parents should inform the family as to who they have chosen to make health care decisions on their behalf so that person, or persons, can be contacted in an emergency. It is important that all family members be aware of your parents' wishes when it comes to resuscitation and extending life through the use of machines, as well as their intentions regarding organ donation. Impress upon your parents that only by being vocal about their wishes can they ensure that in a time of crisis these will be carried out without causing disagreements among the rest of the family. (More information on legal issues can be found in Chapter 7.)

FINANCES

In the event that your parents need to be hospitalized for a short period of time you should be aware of how the regular household bills such as property taxes and car payments are handled. Which ones are paid through automatic withdrawal? What sort of income or payments do your parents receive and what bank accounts are these deposited into? Your parents don't need to reveal details if they are still healthy and active, but they need to understand how important it is for you to know where to find this information if they need to be away from their home for an extended period of time. If anything, this should put their minds at ease.

You should also be aware of where they keep the following:

- bank records
- tax returns
- titles to property and vehicles
- investment information
- retirement information.

If you have not been assigned power of attorney for your parents' property and finances, the person who is responsible should be made aware of your parents' situation and where your parents' information can be found if needed. (Chapter 7 explores this subject in more detail.)

LIVING ARRANGEMENTS AND PERSONAL CARE

How are your parents set up for their retirement? What do they want to do should health concerns result in the need for extended care? Are they comfortable having outside caregivers come into their home to provide personal care if necessary? What are their thoughts on retirement facilities? Do they have enough to live on going forward, and have they made any financial arrangements to cover alternative living arrangements? This could be the most difficult part of the conversation because your parents may not have thought through the various possibilities and may not want to reveal that they are in debt or that their financial situation is precarious. Likely both you and your parents will have to do some research into the various types of facilities available, what they can afford privately, what's covered by your provincial government, and what is available under federal legislation. If you are currently trying to decide what's best for your parents, see Chapter 4, which discusses helping your parents stay in their home, and Chapter 5, which discusses various housing options.

END-OF-LIFE WISHES

Perhaps hardest of all, you need to determine your parents last wishes and what arrangements they want to make in advance for their funeral and burial. This is most commonly what everyone thinks about when they are asked if they have thought about their future. (See Chapter 7 for more details.)

Don't Wait

Have this conversation with your parents while they are still healthy and active! Don't wait until circumstances force you to make hasty decisions that you and your parents might regret. Once you have taken the time to talk with your parents all of you will feel more secure.

Noticing that Your Parents Need Help

As your parents age, your family will start taking on a minor caregiver role. Most often parents first start to need help around the house, for example doing the laundry or cutting the grass. Your visits, which will probably become more frequent, will include finding ways to make their tasks around the house easier (see the Home Safety checklist in Chapter 4 for some suggestions for modifying the home).

If both your parents are alive, you may assume they can take care of each other and do not need your help. You may not realize how much care one parent is providing to the other until a crisis reveals the true situation. Paying attention to such details is key in the early stages.

Frequent communication and personal contact is very important in creating an environment where your parents feel safe talking to you about what is going on in their lives and, eventually, asking you for help. Ask questions about their day, what they had for breakfast or dinner, what their plans are for the week, and really listen to their answers. Be observant and watch for non-verbal signs. That way,

As your parents age, so do you. You always think your parents will be around forever, however, when they are gone, they are gone forever. Cherish each moment you have. When they're gone you will miss the good talks and advice they once gave you. Their living knowledge is the best knowledge. Remember, they know more than you do, because they have lived longer. They are wise and are truly looking after your best interest. Whether you are twelve or fifty-two, you are still their child and they will continue to worry forever. One day you will be the aging parent, so take good care of your aging parents and your children will look after you.

MANON, CORNWALL, ONTARIO

> My husband and I work late and my mom preferred to eat an early dinner. I would call my mom on the way home from work to let her know when I was on the road and to ask her what she was having for supper. I knew it was hard to cook for just one and I think knowing I was going to ask helped motivate my mom to eat. She didn't like to cook as much any more so we had started buying a variety of frozen meals for those nights when she wasn't up to it. She had her favourites and she would supplement them with salads, vegetables and desserts.
>
> LINDA

with luck, you can anticipate problems before they turn into a crisis.

If you notice problems your parents are not willing to share with you, it might be appropriate to talk discreetly to their friends or neighbours. You might learn that a family friend is driving your mom to her regular doctor visits, or that a neighbour takes their trash to the curb each week. Be aware of how much your parents are handling and how this is changing. As our parents age they sometimes believe they can do more than they physically can. Recognizing these changes can prevent a situation that compromises your parents' safety and health.

There are several areas that you can keep an eye on to judge how well your parents are doing and to identify when a situation is intensifying to a point where you need to put structured help in place.

Food Tells You When Help Is Required

Observing your parents' eating habits can help you to gauge how they are doing because food preparation is a daily activity and involves many steps, from buying the food to preparing it to maintaining the kitchen. Food is also crucial to their health and well-being. By talking to your parents about what they are eating you can touch on several important aspects of their lives. For example, have they stopped socializing with their usual network of friends? Are they showing signs of depression? Are they still going out to shop for themselves? How are they handling the tasks required to prepare a meal and clean up afterward? The subject of food is generally a neutral one that can be used as a conversational gateway to other aspects of your parents' lives. For example, as you talk about cooking a simple meal, you may discover that your mom is having trouble opening jars because her arthritis is worsening. If so, you can look at other areas in the house where you can make things simpler for her, given her condition.

But before jumping to conclusions about your parents' eating habits consider that a person's relationship with food changes as they get older. Taste buds are less sensitive so foods taste different and favourite meals may no longer taste so good. A mother who has cooked for a household of people for many years may be leading a very active retirement and may not be interested in cooking any more. Takeout dinners or eating out may have taken the place of home-cooked meals. It is normal for older seniors to have a reduced appetite, and if your parents are living alone they may be less motivated to cook for only themselves.

TELL-TALE SIGNS IN THE KITCHEN

- Do your parents frequently have little or no food in the house?
- Have they had several small accidents with appliances? For example, allowing a coffee pot or kettle to burn dry, or leaving the stove or oven on.
- Do the pots have burn marks on the bottoms?
- Is there spoiled food in the fridge?
- Is the kitchen continually untidy or even unsanitary?

If you answered yes to any of these, talk to your parents about what they are experiencing and see what solutions you can come up with, together, to make it easier for them to eat healthily.

STEPPING IN: DINNER ON THE TABLE

Working with your parents to find solutions to food issues will require some creative thinking. The range of available frozen microwave entrees has increased dramatically in the last few years with new and healthier choices on the market. These are a great alternative for seniors who don't want to be bothered with cooking full meals for themselves or who are having difficulty using the stove.

If your parents are not interested in commercial frozen entrees, another solution might be for you to make extra portions

Where to begin with stories to share about my mother?

Her Alzheimer's condition started with paranoia, not trusting anyone, especially family members, fearful of everything—a very changed woman who once was a strong, witty and powerful lady.

Sadly, my mom made me promise never to send her to a home, "Now promise me that, Lynda!" Of course, I did promise and that promise proved to be the hardest thing in the world to live with, even today.

Lucky for me, I have great sons who always took an interest in their grandmother and a wonderful husband who was there for me every step of the way.

Food was an important issue—she could not cook for herself—but luckily one of my sons came up with a brilliant idea. We would have a cook-off every four to five months, with me and the three men. We would make eight entrees with coordinating veggies and starches. We cooked everything that day, from a roast turkey to lamb chops, lasagna, etc., all her favourites. Then we would portion out the freezer dishes and load up her freezer. She was set for another few months. Plus mom joined us three to four times a week for dinner and loved the company.

LYNDA, MARKHAM, ONTARIO

when you cook for your family, and freeze these in microwave-safe dishes. This way you know that your parents are enjoying healthy meals, because they are eating what you are eating.

Recently new companies have emerged to support busy families, and these companies can also benefit seniors and their caregivers. They provide fresh, pre-prepared food options, which you or your parent can easily cook at home. Some offer the opportunity to cook meals in their facility, allowing you to cook a month's worth of frozen meals without having to do the dishes. Check your local newspaper or the phone book or search online.

STEPPING IN: GROCERY SHOPPING

If going to the grocery store seems too much for your parent physically, look into the world of online shopping. Groceries can be ordered and delivered to your parents' door at their convenience. If there is no online delivery service in your area, you may be able to make arrangements with one of your local grocery stores to set up an account and order by phone for pickup or delivery. If you are not able to be in regular contact with your parents, an option is to make arrangements with an organization such as Meals on Wheels, which provides prepared meals, chosen by your parents, to be delivered to their door. Or, you can investigate other community services in your area.

Meals on Wheels are regionally run volunteer organizations. Search online for Meals on Wheels in your city to find a location near you, or check your telephone directory. Alternatively, contact organizations such as the Canadian Red Cross, the Victorian Order of Nurses, the United Way or the Salvation Army, any of which may offer food delivery services in your community.

If you do live close by, perhaps you could combine your parents' weekly shopping trip with your own. Though grocery shopping is rarely considered an exciting event, it can become a special opportunity for you and your parents to spend time together. It is also a time when you can chat with your parents about other aspects of their daily lives, and perhaps discover other ways in which you need to get involved.

My parents lived in Ottawa and I live in Halifax. When my mother passed away a year and a half ago, I helped my dad move out to Nova Scotia because I am the only family he has left. I am married, but I have no children, and I work full time and have a busy household because I have so many pets to take care of. My father is an octogenarian but does have quite good health and is not disabled, so that makes life somewhat easier.

I pick my father up and take him for groceries. Since he doesn't get out much, this is actually quite an outing for him. I tended to rush through my grocery shopping, viewing it as an evil necessity done on the run. With seniors who don't get out very much and move more slowly, grocery shopping tends to be much more drawn out. For the longest time I would go around with my dad at a snail's pace. I actually found it very difficult to walk as slowly as he does. Now I just let him do his own thing in the store and I pick up my groceries and hover around the magazine section for the duration of the stay, or I browse so long that I end up spending money on things I don't need or can't even afford sometimes! I won't rush him because I know he likes the exercise, and even though it takes him an hour and a half to put about twenty items in his cart, he enjoys getting out. He still hasn't figured out how to buy for one person instead of two. He may never figure that out, but at least he still has the will to eat and go on without his best friend of forty years.

CHRISTINE, HALIFAX, NOVA SCOTIA

When Help Is Required: Housekeeping

If you notice that the kitchen is not being cleaned properly, you may need to do an informal assessment of the house. Keep in mind that as people age their eyesight diminishes, so you are bound to spot the odd place that didn't get dusted or wiped and that is nothing to worry about. But if the house in general is not being cleaned and laundry isn't being done, determine with your parents if housework has become too much for them.

Housecleaning services are widely available. Arranging this can be expensive, but some offer senior discounts, or scales of payment based on service required and income. It may be important to your parents that the same person comes each time, or that the person who comes knows how to interact with seniors. For senior-specific services, contact a local senior organization, which you can find in your telephone directory, or check your municipal website for suggestions. A service might be worth the cost if it allows your parents to remain independent and living in their own home longer.

Some provinces offer a senior's guide to programs and services (consult our Senior and Caregiver Resource Guide under your province). Under the Alberta program, a doctor's note allows for monetary support for yardwork and housekeeping. Quebec has a program that provides for a reduction in fees from approved domestic help companies for services such as light housework, laundry, heavy cleaning, meal preparation and errands. In most provinces, municipalities offer snow-clearing, and garbage and recycling assistance for seniors.

When Help Is Required: Driving, the Hot-Button Issue

The most potentially inflammatory of all discussions with your aging parents has to be about when they should stop driving. Chances are they are going to be the least open and honest with you about their ability to continue driving because the loss

My dad was always the one driving me to places as I was growing up. He took me to school events, Girl Guides and on family trips and never complained. But as the years went by, I started to notice that he was not as alert as he once was behind the wheel. It made me nervous to know he was driving but I was hesitant to bring it up with him. I started to offer to drive, especially long distances, when we had family gatherings. After being involved in two car accidents over a short period of time he eventually decided to give up his licence. I know it was a difficult decision for him but he knew it was for the best. I like the idea that I am now helping my dad get around like he did for me when I was young.

BARBARA

of a car is a huge threat to their independence. Your parents may know deep down that one day they will have to give up driving, but that does not mean they will voluntarily hand over the keys.

This is an emotional issue for our parents because a car gives them autonomy and mobility, and even, for some, self-esteem and personal identity. When our parents have to give up driving, they know they will need to rely on others to get around and will feel restricted in their activities.

Some people can't depend on public transportation. Some parents may not be able to walk to a bus stop or may find public transit too confusing. Or public transportation may not get them where they want to go quickly enough, or at all. When we discuss this issue with our parents, we need to recognize why they would want to continue to drive as long as possible, so that we can show empathy.

HOW TO KNOW WHEN DRIVING IS BECOMING A CHALLENGE

If your parents keep their concerns a secret, how do you know that driving has become dangerous for them? Unfortunately, you won't know unless your parents mention that they are nervous behind the wheel, or can't see well enough any more, or have had several near misses or a minor accident. In some cases you'll

SENIORS' DRIVING HABITS

You may notice your aging parents starting to modify their driving habits by

- driving to familiar places only by regular routes
- avoiding highways
- staying closer to home
- driving less at night
- avoiding driving in bad weather.

As a caregiver you can

- encourage your parents to plan routes for new destinations
- hold family events early in the day
- offer to drive them places
- encourage them to change or cancel appointments in bad weather
- encourage them to talk to their doctor or pharmacist about how their medications may affect their driving.

know only when your parents receive a doctor's diagnosis that clearly tells them it's time to give up the keys.

If you do have an open dialogue with your parents, they may tell you the issues they are facing with driving. Perhaps these are specific to certain conditions, such as driving after dark, or driving on the highway, or driving long distances. To help them avoid these situations, and so that they drive less frequently, you can offer to be available to drive them for errands, appointments or family gatherings.

Understanding how aging affects driving skills will help you identify when driving is becoming a challenge for your parents. The physical constraints of aging may arise from problems with vision (depth perception, peripheral vision, night vision), physical ability (range of motion, pain in legs and arms), reaction time, hearing or medication. A parent who is starting to have difficulties in these areas may not necessarily have to give up the keys to the car right away. With your help they may be able to adjust their driving habits in a positive way that will allow them to continue to drive for a few more years.

STEPPING IN: ASKING YOUR PARENTS TO GIVE UP THE KEYS

Be warned that even if your parents are adjusting their driving habits themselves it is unlikely that they will admit that's what they are doing. Instead you may hear that they don't have the same interest in road trips any more, or that their friends are all close by so why would they need to venture farther, or that the price of gas or limited retirement funds is keeping them close to home. All these things may in fact be true, but it's unlikely that you will hear, "I'm not seeing as well as I used to," or "I find the number of cars and speed overwhelming."

A note of caution: do not jump to the wrong conclusion and demand that keys be turned over if your aging parent has a car accident. Sometimes a car accident is just a car accident—something that could have happened to anyone. If you realize that your parents are having an increased number of near misses, however, or if they have been involved in several accidents, it might be time to address the issues directly.

If your parents have been in an accident, even if no other car was involved, the rules of your province may require that their driving skills be re-evaluated. Also, if they have been diagnosed with a significant health condition (diabetes, heart problems or dementia), you will need to know how these may affect their abilities and whether their doctor has advised them to stop driving. In most provinces, doctors are required to report to the licensing authorities any patient who is unfit to drive due to medical conditions. A doctor's report to the licensing authority can result in a person needing to take a driver's test or having his or her licence suspended.

If your parents feel that they would like to take a refresher course or have their driving skills evaluated, you can contact a local driving school or an organization such as the Canadian Automobile Association (CAA), both of which offer driver improvement courses. Some senior centres also sponsor programs to improve seniors' driving skills.

If you are concerned about your parents' driving skills, arrange to be a passenger the next time they drive or suggest that you will follow them. This will allow you to gauge their current ability. You may want to do this regularly in order to judge whether their skills are worsening.

See our Senior and Caregiver Resource Guide for provincial Ministry of Transportation websites that offer seniors driving tips.

If you do find yourself having to talk to your parents about giving up driving, be sure to pick a suitable time and have the conversation in private. Understand that your parents may not react well to having their physical abilities questioned and their source of independence threatened. Help them recognize that due to medical or physical changes beyond their control it is no longer safe for them to drive. Try to make them understand that you are concerned for their safety and the safety of others on the road.

If your parents have been diagnosed with a progressive medical condition, discuss with your parents what they will do when they reach the stage that they can't drive. Begin this dialogue early, before the situation becomes a crisis.

STEPPING IN: ALTERNATIVES TO DRIVING

When talking to your parents about the issue of driving it's helpful to discuss alternatives. For example, you could arrange to set up an account with a local taxi company. This way your parents might get to know a regular driver or dispatcher, which would give them confidence in who is driving them. Alternatively, there are volunteer driving programs available in most communities; some are free and some charge based on distance travelled or on income. Another option is to have a family member drive your parents' car for them. This way the car remains with your parents and they allow others to act as chauffeur, but be sure to investigate insurance implications. This could be an opportunity to allow young people in the family the time to bond with the older generation.

Suggesting alternatives to driving shows that you understand the significance of your parents giving up the car and reinforces that you want to help them maintain their independence.

Volunteer transportation for seniors can be found by contacting local senior centres and services. Some not-for-profit organizations also provide this service.

If your parents just won't cooperate in giving up driving, you may need to look to a third party for help. Sometimes hearing the truth from someone else, especially a professional, can convince them in a way that a dialogue within the family cannot. In the end, if your parents are having minor accidents, their insurance company may make their decision for them. And in most provinces when your parents reach eighty years old they need to be retested in order to keep their licences.

The Importance of Social Networks

Mental and emotional health has a direct impact on our parents' physical health. It's natural for them to develop some health problems as they get older, but feelings of self-worth and connectedness to the world play a significant role in how they age. Today's seniors enjoy a longer period of good health and active living than any generation before them; it is during

In the report "A Portrait of Seniors in Canada," the Canadian government identified a positive outlook on life as critical to the well-being of seniors.[10]

these years that you should encourage your parents to develop hobbies, get involved with their communities and maintain and establish social networks. If our parents can remain active and interested in the world around them, they will stay young of mind and light of heart.

As seniors age their risk of social isolation increases. They eventually start to lose friends and family, even their spouse, leaving them with an increasingly smaller social circle. Parents who are housebound and reliant on family and neighbours for social contact can develop difficulties with their health. For seniors in this stage, you and your family may have to take an active role in re-establishing a social network. If your parents are still driving or able to travel, look for community courses that they might be interested in, afternoon lectures to attend or clubs to join. As well, volunteering is a positive way for your parents to feel that they are contributing to their community, one that helps to promote feelings of self-esteem and self-worth.

Your local community centre may have senior programs or you may have senior centres in your area. You can locate these through your local telephone directory or your municipal office, or by searching online.

The Internet is a quick and easy way for them to keep in contact with family and friends, via e-mail and webcam, and to keep up with world news and community happenings. It's also an invaluable tool that allows seniors to order food, entertainment, clothes and other products, and renew prescriptions. If your parents are not online yet, what are you waiting for? This is an opportunity to teach your parents something new.

Several years ago I decided I wanted to set aside time to spend with my mom. I have always had a good relationship with her and usually talked to her every day on the phone. I looked around and decided that a gardening club would be the answer. My mom loves roses and had a beautiful garden that reflects her abilities. The meetings were once a month and it was something we both enjoyed.

My father's health started to deteriorate and we decided that in order for him to move to an assisted living environment, we needed to sell their home. This decision was extremely difficult for Mom. She had always talked about fixing up the back room and having a picture window that looked out at her garden. It never happened. Mom moved in with my younger sister and her family. They have provided a loving environment for her but for Mom it took months before she did not feel like a guest in their home. I was busy looking after my father and trying to get him settled into his new home and making sure we had his health problems under control. I knew that my mother was being well looked after. I did not have much time to spend with her and the travelling time prevented Mom and me from attending the garden club meetings.

My sister's home was in a new development in Oakville and she suggested Mom might enjoy having a garden again. This was a great idea. My husband and I headed over to their place with a carload of gardening supplies and attacked the soil. Even before we had it ready Mom had pots of plants waiting for their new home. The garden is her place to retreat. She may not remember the names of all the plants but she knows what a garden can do for your soul.

JOAN, TORONTO, ONTARIO

If your parents are in their older senior years and not as active as they used to be, look into more structured programs or environments that allow them to connect with people their own age. Programs that provide day programs or periodic activities are available through local community centres, churches and cultural organizations. As well, some private organizations run day programs for seniors.

Before seeking out programs for your parents, take into consideration their personalities. If they never liked playing cards or being involved in big social gatherings when they were young, they likely aren't going to take to it now. Don't try to force your parents into activities that you think they should enjoy—instead provide them with options. If you or another family member has time, find something you can do with your parents so that they don't have to go alone.

In my mom's early senior years she re-established a relationship with music and started studying the piano. As a young person she'd played, and in her retirement she decided to take it up again. The study, not just the playing of the instrument, gave her something that challenged her mind. She said quite often how it enriched her life.

She had a wonderful music teacher who arranged grand soirées where the adult students performed. Having attended one of these evenings with my mom I saw that she was surrounded by an interesting and passionate group of music lovers, who cared for and respected her. My mom talked about her hobby with enthusiasm and passion—and she spent hours on the computer monitoring music forums with other students and music teachers.

LINDA

There may eventually be health reasons that require you to find a day program for your parents, whether it's because they can't stay at home by themselves or because you are providing twenty-four-hour care and need a break yourself.

Senior day programs provide a place for seniors to spend the day in a supervised environment. Often they offer activities, social opportunities and meals, and in some cases, limited health services. You can find one by contacting your local senior centre or not-for-profit organizations in your community. For seniors with specific medical needs, your local hospital can provide you with information.

Communicating with your parents is vital if you are to know whether they are suffering from depression, or feeling isolated or lonely. Parents in their senior years will experience not only loss of family and friends but also loss of independence, and of physical and mental ability. Ultimately they are facing their mortality. We should treat our parents with love and respect, recognizing that we still have much to learn from them and that they still have a great deal to offer our families and our community.

Knowing When to Take Action

We have talked about recognizing signs of aging and becoming involved with our parents in the early stages. However, there may come a time when you are forced to take more definitive action to ensure your parents' safety and long-term well-being.

Specialists who work not only in the field of gerontology but in many different clinical and rehabilitation settings use two systems of assessment to determine how well a person is able to function within their personal space and in the community. These systems also help to determine what level of care your parents require. One is called Instrumental Activities of Daily Living (IADL) and the other is called Activities of Daily Living (ADL).

INSTRUMENTAL ACTIVITIES OF DAILY LIVING (IADL)

An assessment of the Instrumental Activities of Daily Living indicates how well individuals are functioning. Even though your parents may need some assistance or require someone to take on full responsibility in certain areas of their lives, they are still able to function around the home and within the community with a high degree of independence. How much assistance they need is often difficult to gauge; it requires keen observation during visits and constructive communication.

INSTRUMENTAL ACTIVITIES OF DAILY LIVING

Consider the following to determine whether your parents need some help but are still able to live independently. Can they

- prepare their own meals?
- go shopping?
- perform basic tasks around the house (laundry, housekeeping)?
- drive or use other transportation?
- manage their finances?
- manage their medications?
- care for pets and others?

Adapted from Rehabilitation Services, "Rehabilitation Standard: Instrumental Activities of Daily Living (IADL)," Vancouver Island Health Authority, 2006.

ACTIVITIES OF DAILY LIVING (ADL)

Your parents must be able to perform Activities of Daily Living self-care functions in order to live on their own and without assistance. If you answer yes to one or more of the questions below then your parent is no longer safe living alone. You must take action.

ACTIVITIES OF DAILY LIVING

The following are signs that your parents are no longer able to live on their own. Are they

- experiencing continence problems?
- unable to feed themselves?
- unable to perform personal hygiene (washing or bathing)?
- unable to perform toileting functions by themselves?
- unable to dress themselves?
- unable to perform general mobility functions such as getting in and out of bed, or on and off a chair or toilet, or using the phone?

Adapted from Rehabilitation Services, "Rehabilitation Standard: Self Care (ADL)," Vancouver Island Health Authority, 2006.

If your parents are unable to perform some or all of these self-care functions, recognize that there is a crisis at hand and assess the situation quickly to determine the next course of action.

How do you know whether your parents are experiencing difficulties performing critical functions? Signs to watch for are changes in

- socialization: withdrawing from family, suddenly stopping activities they once enjoyed
- personal hygiene: wearing the same clothes over and over, or exhibiting body odour
- eating habits: suddenly losing weight; or keeping too little food or spoiled food in the house
- approach to finances: not paying bills, not opening mail

- approach to taking medication: leaving loose pills around the house; being disorganized or confused about taking medications
- mobility: having difficulty walking, exhibiting unexplained bruises, having frequent accidents
- mental ability: exhibiting short-term memory loss, showing confusion, being unable to perform routine tasks, or frequently getting lost.

If you notice any of these signs, notify your family doctor to have him or her assess your parents' physical and mental health. A geriatric assessment (covered in detail in Chapter 6) will help to determine the type of health care services your parents need.

You are now communicating with your parents as a caregiver. You are asking them to look at you in a new role. You are no longer just their child but a trusted adult helping them to make decisions that will affect their lives and your family. In the next chapter, we explore family dynamics, and the importance of keeping the lines of communication among family members open in order to make the best decisions with our parents.

3

FAMILY DYNAMICS

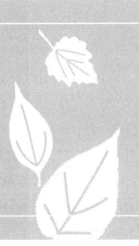

In most cases, if you ask, you'll likely find that the role of caregiver is taken on by a family member quietly and slowly if no health crisis demands immediate action. You may have taken on this new role yourself, without really understanding how it was going to impact your relationship with your siblings, extended family and immediate family. This chapter will address

- the reasons for conflict within families
- steps for conflict-resolution
- the family meeting and other methods to keep in touch with the extended family
- communicating with your partner and children about your parents' changing needs.

Conflict Due to Differing Personalities

Within all families, members have varying approaches toward communication and abilities to work together. Caregiving for your parents doesn't involve just your siblings, but sometimes your parents' own siblings or extended family members, and even friends. When you take on the role of caregiver, you need to make decisions and take charge and this may result in conflict in the family. Everyone will have an opinion on what you do and the decisions you make. As a caregiver already struggling with decisions big and small, this constant questioning of your choices can create added frustration and stress.

Everyone in the family may have a different view of how things should be done, so communication needs to be fostered to avoid hurt feelings. Understand that each person has his or her own personal strengths and abilities, and allow people to take on different caregiving roles for your parents. There are many tasks and responsibilities; if willing, everyone in the family can be involved in some way.

Within a family you have not only a variety of beliefs and values but also a range of personalities. For example, the critical person may now critique the quality of care; the person who can't make a decision in their own life may now dither when one has to be made for your parents; the person who agrees to everything, thinking they are being supportive when they are actually leaving the tough decision-making to others, may do the same when it comes to your parents; or the person who doesn't tend to participate may stay out of discussions but then question decisions. The complexity of personalities and issues creates strained relationships and increased stress.

Conflict arises when two people with differing interpretations of a situation enter into a must-win combat. Instead of looking for a compromise, or trying to understand each other's perspective, they engage in a battle of wills. When these conflicts arise, parents and children are hurt by the fighting and mistrust, all family members suffer stress and guilt, and ultimately attention is diverted from the main issue: quality of care for your parents.

Conflict Due to Perception of Need

At the root of most caregiving conflicts is a difference in opinion over the senior's needs. One family member may feel that the situation is not as bad as others are portraying it, and therefore they do not want to take immediate action or consider a long-term solution. For example, a caregiver may believe that their aging parents can no longer live alone in the house and wants to make alternative living arrangements, but a sibling believes that the family just needs to visit the parents more often.

The conflict over perceived needs can occur in both the

My mother-in-law, who had lived independently, had surgery that required assisted recovery. She stayed with me for the first month after she was out of hospital, even though her son, my husband, worked out of town. Though her daughter lived very close by, she stayed with me because our house had no stairs. With my husband away and no children living at home, she knew I would wait on her—cook for her, help her to shower, and drive her to physio. But once she was well enough to climb stairs she couldn't wait to leave our place—she went to stay with her daughter. In quick order, her daughter convinced her to sell her house and move in with her family. But they made no concessions for her; she had no say in meals, TV channels, visitors, etc. She had no TV or phone in her room, and she had to climb up stairs to her room and down stairs to do laundry. She was expected to buy groceries. But she stayed anyway.

Eventually my brother-in-law decided that he had enough—he no longer wanted his mother-in-law with them and gave her marching orders. She no longer had a house to return to, and no financial means to go into any type of senior complex without assistance from us. She has a sister who lives a distance away, but she cried to my husband on the phone that she would be homeless, and he felt he had no option but to allow her to stay with us.

CAREGIVER, KELOWNA, BRITISH COLUMBIA

FAMILY DYNAMICS

small and the big decisions that are made during successive stages of parents' aging. For the caregiver, these disputes can result in them feeling responsible for the lion's share of the work, and unappreciated.

Conflict Resulting from Family History

As our relationships were when we were children, so they continue as we grow up. It often happens that adult children who are able to relate to one another at family functions in a mature and friendly way regress to the squabbling siblings of childhood during a time of family crisis. Suddenly the sibling who you feel was always considered the rational one is being asked to make decisions, while you are the one devoting time to caring for your aging parent. Old rivalries and past hurts become the basis from which all your problem solving originates, hindering clear judgment and decision-making.

Poor sibling relations are not the only causes of conflict. Once the extended family is involved in the caregiving discussion, family histories play a role as well. While it generally is beneficial to include in the decision-making everyone who is affected by caregiving for your parents, in some situations, to avoid strife, there may be certain family members who should be on a need-to-know list.

Conflict Due to Dysfunctional Relationships

If you didn't have a loving relationship with your parents prior to their needing you to take on a caregiving role it may be difficult at this late stage to foster one. Your role may therefore have its basis in obligation and duty rather than devotion and commitment. As a result you might approach each decision and act of help with feelings of anger.

It is unrealistic to believe that any family functions without some conflicts. But the family that is truly dysfunctional, that cannot support its members and fosters a negative environment, will struggle tremendously if they have to come together to make caregiving decisions for their parents.

Parent-to-Parent Relationships as a Barrier to Caregiving

If you are dealing with both parents as they age, there are often added areas of conflict. Some aspects of your parents' relationship are private and how they relate to each other and the past they share can manifest itself in ways that make caregiving harder. For example, one parent may be ill and receiving extra attention from the family and this may cause feelings of resentment in the other parent. Or perhaps the parent who is not in medical crisis has a history of sacrificing for the family and doesn't mention his or her own medical needs. Or perhaps all the children believe that one parent is taking care of the other and so no one steps in to ensure that proper decisions are being made or adequate care is being given. Often as children we feel it isn't our place to be involved in the dynamics between our parents. Unfortunately, in some cases this means our aging parents don't receive the help that is needed and conflicts can arise.

> I walked in to my father-in-law's room and immediately I thought he doesn't really want me here, after all I am family, and a woman to boot, and in his eyes a woman should not be caring for a man. But since that evening we have formed a special bond together, a different level of respect, understanding and trust. And knowing that he trusts me to care for him completely amazes me. He is truly a unique person and it is this quality I have come to admire in him.
>
> MARIEANNE, LAKEVILLE, NEW BRUNSWICK

Solving Conflict

How does a family come together and work their way through the conflicts that can interfere with good decision-making to reach the ultimate goal of

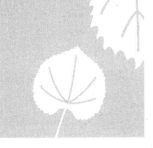

- different opinions of what should be done
- different values and beliefs used to evaluate situations
- different personalities
- differences in perceived need
- family history
- selfish motives
- desire to win, not to compromise

providing the best care for the parents? Removing the win-or-lose aspect of the problem is key to finding resolution. Use the steps below as a guide for initiating a problem-solving dialogue. These steps can be used when trying to find solutions for big or small issues, with a group or one-on-one.

STEP 1: IDENTIFY THE PROBLEM

Clearly identify the problem that is causing conflict. Ensure that everyone understands and agrees what's at issue. Determine why it is a problem and who is affected. What will be the result if the problem isn't resolved?

STEP 2: TALK ABOUT THE PROBLEM

Have anyone who is affected by the problem express feelings about it. Everyone should share how he or she feels the current situation affects them. This reveals the shared issues and conflicting perceptions around the problem.

Allow each person to speak uninterrupted without fear of accusation or reprisal. Be considerate of other's feelings. Listen actively.

STEP 3: SHARE SOLUTIONS

Have everyone participating in the problem solving share ideas for solutions. Create an open environment where everyone is given the opportunity to speak and no idea is rejected. At this stage you are just looking for everyone's thoughts. By allowing everyone to contribute you will find they are better committed to the final resolution.

STEP 4: RATE SOLUTIONS

After everyone has been allowed to put forward ideas, the next step is to review and rate them in terms of how they best satisfy the needs of your parents and other family members.

STEP 5: DECIDE ON A RESOLUTION

To find a resolution you need to be flexible and creative. Perhaps one solution stands out as the best. Or, by taking a couple of the best options and breaking these down into pros and cons, you may find a good solution. Perhaps combining parts of different ideas will result in an acceptable solution. Or it could be that you arrive at only a temporary solution. If so, problems can be revisited down the road to make sure that the temporary solutions are still working for family members who were affected, or who became involved through the resolution.

On the other hand, at this stage it might be determined that a resolution can't be found in the ideas presented, in which case research into other options will need to be done and brought back to another discussion.

STEP 6: BE CLEAR ABOUT THE RESOLUTION

Make sure the solution has been stated clearly and that everyone understands it and acknowledges the consequences of the decision.

These steps for working through problems may not work for you and your family. If they don't, another way to proceed might be to hire a professional mediator or contact a social services agency to come in and help assess and mediate problems as they arise. If the situation is critical to the health and well-being of your aging parents, then as the caregiver you may need to make a quick decision on your own and deal with the family repercussions later.

A Role for Everyone

Now that you know your parents need help and you have identified yourself as a caregiver, the next step is to assemble the family and discuss honestly the roles that people are able or willing to take on. The goal is to determine who is able to participate, what expertise is available, and what commitment people are willing to make, based on the current situation and into the future.

> I have a big family (two sisters and three brothers) but I was the only one who had the time to look after our mother and schedule my life around her appointments. Not once did I realize the toll it was going to take on my life. As the weeks turned into months and the months turned into years, the workload has only gotten larger.
>
> GLYNIS, BRANTFORD, ONTARIO

Figuring out roles for each member of the family can help prevent conflict. Caregiving may require years of involvement and to help cope as a family you will need to put systems in place for efficient communication and problem solving. One of the tools you can use is the modern concept of the family meeting.

The Family Meeting

The goal of the family meeting is, first and foremost, to focus on the needs of your aging parents. As we discuss elsewhere in this book, the role of the family is to listen to your parents and to help them retain their independence and personal dignity as they move

> We had to have our first family meeting after a dramatic change in my dad's behaviour. We had to figure out what the next steps were: where would Mom and Dad live? What did we need to research and do? It was also to update everyone so they were aware of everything that had happened. I had my doubts that it would actually be useful.
>
> I remember walking into my sister's house and, as I was getting some breakfast from the table, joking about having a family meeting. We must all have been a bit anxious, as we chuckled at my comment even though it wasn't really that funny.
>
> The meeting was a good chance for everyone to give opinions and offer what help they could. Some of us were given tasks and some of us did more research. In the end it seemed to work, and it was important to connect face-to-face in the midst of a crisis.
>
> BARBARA

through the various stages of aging. The family meeting's second goal is to support the caregiver and other members of the family who are taking on helping roles. Such a meeting will be a success only if solutions are found to meet your parents' needs and if the caregiver receives the support and help he or she needs.

The family meeting ensures some level of communication among those responsible for the aging parents, finds solutions to care issues, assigns responsibilities and garners commitments from family members, helps prevent family members who are self-motivated from making care decisions out of their own interest, and provides a forum for conflict resolution.

If you adopt the family meeting structure as your means of communication and making decisions, avoid clandestine meetings that might cause bad feelings among your family or

Here are some tips for family meetings:

- Include everyone who is affected by caregiving decisions, including your parents.
- Decide how you are going to communicate with family who live out of town and include them in the discussions.
- Select a day for the initial meeting and proceed with whoever can attend. Set subsequent meeting dates so that people can calendar them.
- Have an agenda with specific topics for each meeting.
- Set a time limit for each meeting.
- Establish rules for the meeting allowing uninterrupted times to speak and good behaviour guidelines.
- Secure and record commitments from family members.
- Take minutes and distribute among family.

Select a chairperson who will keep the meeting moving and ensure everyone minds their manners. A good chairperson is able to

- take control of the meeting without dominating the discussion
- keep the meeting focused
- keep the meeting moving, conscious of the allotted time
- ensure everyone has a chance to talk
- ensure everyone minds their manners
- be well organized and follow an agenda
- be a good mediator.

The family meeting is a success if the needs of the aging parents are met and the caregiver is provided with support.

chance alienating your parents. You will defeat the purpose of the family meeting.

If Family Meetings Aren't for You

The family meeting structure won't work for everyone. In Barbara's situation, with five sisters and two brothers, the family meeting was used initially to make key decisions and set the basic care structures in place. Down the road additional family meetings might be called, but for now they have found other ways to communicate and make decisions.

For Linda there was no extended family to involve—only her mother, husband and brother—so formal meetings were not required. It was understood that Linda was the primary caregiver and would work directly with her mom to make decisions, involving others along the way as needed.

If family meetings don't fit into your family dynamic, try a more casual form of communication. If your family talks often anyway and you all communicate well, use these discussions as opportunities to touch base on how things are going with your parents, or for the caregiver. If your family often disagrees, however, or if there has been miscommunication in the past, give the family meeting a try.

> If family members don't live nearby, you can arrange to have them participate by telephone or Internet conferencing.

In a large family, communication trees can be established. These involve a chain of communication, whereby one person communicates to another, and then each of those people has an assigned person to call to share the information. The communication tree is especially useful in the event of an emergency when the caregiver can't personally call every family member. The phone is a tool that can be used for discussions through conference calling as well.

Keeping family informed may require some creative thinking and exploration of alternatives. Whatever method you set up, ensure that it neither excludes your parents nor adds to the caregiver's burden.

Communication with Your Partner

As the primary caregiver, you likely will have more than just yourself to consider when making decisions about the time you are able to spend looking after your parents. You need to sit down with your spouse or partner to talk about what is happening with your parents and how you feel you want things to proceed and how your involvement will affect your relationship with your immediate family.

While you recognize that decisions need to be made based on what is best for your parents, you also have to come to terms with what you are willing to sacrifice in your life to carry through on those decisions. If you have a partner who is not supportive at all of a situation where your parent needs extensive care, what do you do? What sort of compromise can be made without endangering your parents? We like to think that our partners will be there to support us in these difficult times, but when the situation with our parents could go on for years he or she may feel it's too much to ask. The lack of support of a partner could result in you not being the caregiver, or in you having to find care solutions that involve more formal care options for your parents.

You and your partner may be in a situation where both sets of parents need caregiving. You may be spending time making decisions and running errands for both your parents and your partner's parents. If this is the case, then you may find yourselves depending more on extended family and outside help than if you had just a single parent to consider.

As I thought about caregiving for my parents, I realized that men caregive differently than women do. Sometimes what men contribute is a bit invisible as we women hurry around trying to do everything.

I have watched my husband, Ian, and his brothers and sisters look after their parents. His parents had the foresight to have six children: three boys and three girls, which makes things easier as we all can share the load. His dad who is eighty-nine has Alzheimer's and his mom at eighty-eight looks after the house and keeps his life organized, which puts a lot of pressure on her and keeps her housebound. She knows that her husband has always been a very proud man and would accept help with certain things from his sons but not his daughters. Mom calls her sons for things that her husband would normally have done that he finds too difficult now, like fixing the furnace. When one of the boys goes over, they do things with Dad so he feels included and supported and not replaced in the role that has always been his. When Dad lost his driver's licence, it was the boys who dealt with selling the car and involved Dad in on the decisions. Losing his licence was really hard for him.

Dad's world is narrow. He does better with routine and so prefers to stay at home. However, Mom desperately needs to get out into the bigger world. Therefore the girls take Mom out and the boys do guy things with Dad, like putter in the garage or the garden and talk about guy stuff like cars and machines and fixing things around the house. That way both parents are supported and his mom feels comfortable going out knowing that her husband is cared for.

If we, as women, think that caregiving only works the way we do it, we are missing out on a lot of support. Encouraging men to caregive in their own way is a win-win for all. It allows the men to do more, it helps maintain their parent-son relationships and lessens our load as well. It also makes the boys feel good that they can contribute.

PAT, COOKSTOWN, ONTARIO

FAMILY DYNAMICS

Whatever the situation, it is important that you and your spouse communicate about the status of your parents, what you would like to be able to do and what kind of support you need.

Until you are well into the role of caregiver, you may not have a true sense of the commitment you are making. You will need to have ongoing communication with your partner as your caregiving responsibilities change. You may need to recognize that you and your partner caregive in different ways and learn how to benefit from each other's strengths.

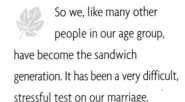

So we, like many other people in our age group, have become the sandwich generation. It has been a very difficult, stressful test on our marriage.

CAREGIVER, KELOWNA, BRITISH COLUMBIA

Your taking on the role of caregiver could be a major strain on your relationship and you may find yourself having to deal with your partner's own feelings of being neglected, or frustration of having to take on responsibility around the house and with the kids. Talking ahead of time and knowing how your partner is going to react will help you to set up any additional support systems you need at home to help you fulfill the responsibility you have taken on for your parents.

Communication with Your Children

In the early stages of caregiving for your parents, your children may not be directly affected by your responsibilities. As your parents' needs increase, your children may start to recognize that you are not available for them as much as before. They may also pick up on any anxiety and stress that results from your caregiving role. Children will react in different ways depending on their age and how you communicate with them about the situation. You should communicate honestly with them about what is going on and why things may change in all your lives.

The conversation should be age appropriate, but even young children will be aware of changes in routine. It is important not to try and hide what is happening. They may be expected to take on more responsibility around the house or be with you when you are carrying out your caregiving tasks. This can be a positive time in your child's life as you teach him or her about family commitment and values. The lessons your children learn about taking on responsibility, communication, family loyalty and ultimately about loving and having compassion for others will be invaluable.

Positive Growth for the Family

Focusing on the negative aspects of caregiving is natural, because there's no question that it's emotionally and physically difficult. But we need to recognize that as we face these hardships we are creating the fabric of our lives. This time with our aging parents gives us the opportunity to create stronger bonds with our family as we grow, learn and share with them.

One benefit of working together for the good of parents is that we can develop closer relationships with our siblings. As adults, busy with our own lives, we don't always stay connected with our sisters and brothers. Often we shift our emotional ties to our spouses and children and lose some of the closeness that we felt with our family growing up. Having to discuss and find workable solutions while caught up in the serious matter of our parents' aging allows us to reconnect on a deeper level with siblings. As you share this mutual experience, you may discover what your siblings are capable of, and gain a new respect and understanding for them.

Grandparents and Children: Building the Bond

If you already encourage a close relationship between your children and their grandparents, you are on the road to providing

Books are available for various age groups that have stories dealing with many common situations around grandparents aging or developing health problems:

- *I'm Going to Grandma's* (ages preschool to 6 years) by Mary Ann Hoberman and illustrated by Tiphanie Beeke (Harcourt Inc., 2007). Summary: A special quilt keeps a little girl from feeling homesick when she sleeps over with her grandparents.
- *Our Granny* (ages preschool to 5 years) by Margaret Wild and illustrated by Julie Vivas (Houghton Mifflin Company, 1993). Summary: While grannies come in all shapes and sizes, "our granny" is unique.
- *Nana Upstairs & Nana Downstairs* (ages 3 to 7 years) by Tomie dePaola (Puffin Books, 1973). Summary: Four-year-old Tommy enjoys his relationship with both his grandmother and his great-grandmother but eventually learns to face their inevitable death.
- *Mile-High Apple Pie* (ages 4 to 6 years) by Laura Langston and illustrated by Lindsey Gardiner (Red Fox, 2005). Summary: A wonderfully moving account of a girl coming to terms with her grandmother not remembering.
- *My Grandparents Are Special* (ages 4 to 7 years) by Jennifer Moore-Mallinos and illustrated by Marta Fabrega (Barrons' Educational Series, 2006). Summary: A warm-hearted story of a child and his grandparents.
- *Now One Foot, Now the Other* (ages 4 to 7 years) by Tomie dePaola (Puffin Books, 2005). Summary: When his grandfather suffers a stroke, Bobby teaches him to walk, just as his grandfather had once taught him.
- *When I Am Old with You* (ages 4 to 7 years) by Angela Johnson and illustrated by David Soman (Orchard Books, 1990). Summary: A child imagines being old with grandaddy and joining him in such activities as playing cards all day, visiting the ocean and eating bacon on the porch.

- *My Little Grandmother Often Forgets* (ages 4 to 8 years) by Reeve Lindbergh and illustrated by Kehtryn Brown (Candlewick Press, 2007). Summary: The story of a special bond between a beloved grandmother affected by memory loss and her patient, devoted grandson.
- *Wilfrid Gordon McDonald Partridge* (ages 4 to 8 years) by Mem Fox and illustrated by Julie Vivas (Kane/Miller Book Publishers, 1989). Summary: A small boy tries to discover the meaning of "memory" so he can restore that of an elderly friend.
- *What's Happening to Grandpa?* (ages 4 to 9 years) by Maria Shriver and illustrated by Sandra Speidel (Little Brown and Company, 2004). Summary: A story of a young girl's acceptance of her grandpa's Alzheimer's.
- *Sunshine Home* (ages 7 to 9 years) by Eve Bunting and illustrated by Diane De Groat (Clarion Books, 1994). Summary: When he and his parents visit his grandmother in the nursing home where she is recovering from a broken hip, everyone pretends to be happy until Tim helps them express their true feelings.
- *The Memory Box* (ages 7 to 11 years) by Mary Bahr and illustrated by David Cunningham (Albert Whitman & Company, 1992). Summary: When Gramps realizes he has Alzheimer's disease, he starts a memory box with his grandson, Zach, to keep memories of all the times they have shared.
- *The Gramma War* (ages 9 to 12 years) by Kristin Butcher (Orca Book Publishers, 2001). Summary: A heartwarming story about change in a young person's life and how she handles it when her gramma moves in.
- *Runaway Gran* (ages 9 to 13 years) by Sonia Craddock (James Lorimer & Company, 2006). Summary: A touching true story about a loved one dealing with dementia and how various family members are affected.

them emotional and psychological benefits that will help them as they grow and stay with them into adulthood.

Grandparents often provide undivided, nonjudgmental attention that helps children build self-esteem and independence. Children who are involved with their grandparents up to and including the stages requiring caregiving also learn to interact with and have a sense of compassion for the elderly, the handicapped and others in need of special care.

Sharing Personal History

One of the most important benefits of spending this time with your parents is giving them the opportunity to share with you and their grandchildren their personal history. As your parents get older you'll notice how often they try to tell you stories about their past. Through these oral histories, they are sharing with you what life has meant to them, and what they have learned along the way—a precious gift.

We can encourage our parents to share of themselves (even if the storytelling happens at frustrating moments). During times of major change or decision-making, your parents may revisit the past as a way to

"Knock, knock."

"Who's there?"

"Banana."

"Banana who?"

"Knock, knock."

"Who's there?"

"Banana."

"Banana who?"

"Knock, knock."

"Who's there?"

"Orange. Orange you glad it's not a banana?"

My three-year-old son is a little comedian. He loves to tell jokes and do funny things. I see my dad in him. My dad is in a retirement home with the early stages of Alzheimer's disease. My dad has a great sense of humour. It's the thing I remember the most about him when I was growing up. He doesn't laugh as much now. But I see his humour come out through my son. I think my dad gets a chuckle once in a while when he hears my son's stories.

CAREGIVER, OAKVILLE, ONTARIO

I couldn't think of anything I wanted to do more than to give my parents the love, devotion, caring, time to listen, and anything they requested in their last months of life. I went from being a daughter to being a friend, and then a nurse. I listened to every word that they spoke. Most of their memories were of the earlier days; how I relished all the wonderful stories that I had never heard before. I began to see these two people who were once my towers of strength and my comfort zones become fragile and weak. I began to realize that I was now the one to give, rather than to receive. The one with the strength, even though at times, I felt like falling apart. That my parents were now depending on *me*, and I would give in every way, for as long as it took, knowing that I could never repay them for all they did for me growing up. I had so little time, and so much to do!

Every day, I see individuals with their elderly parents, shopping, or walking in the park, and I think to myself how blessed they are to still have their parents, but I also think of how blessed I was to have had the opportunity to have given to them peace of mind, comfort, and unconditional love when they needed it most.

Mom and Dad, thank you for making me the person I am today. I love you.

NANCY, CALEDON, ONTARIO

come to terms with the present. It's important to remember, amid the frustration and high emotions, that you are caring for your parents, and the grandparents of your children, and that's a good thing to do and something in which we can find joy.

My grandmother always enjoyed sending Christmas cards. She sent them to a detailed list of friends and family, year after year, until she had a diabetic stroke and couldn't do it any longer. My grandfather took up the task with meticulous care, signing both of their names.

The first Christmas after my grandfather died my grandmother was in a nursing home. I was determined to make Christmas happy and memorable for both of us, so a few weeks before Christmas I went to visit, arms filled with a small Christmas tree, decorations, cards, and (of course) the well-looked-after list of names and addresses.

We spent a lovely afternoon decorating the little tree, carefully placing each ornament, looping strands of gold garland and sparkling silver tinsel until the tree had a personality of its own. Full of Christmas spirit, I pulled out the cards, hopeful that we would be able to make them all out before my grandmother got too tired.

We sat, side-by-side on the bed, while I explained who each card was for and helped guide her hand slowly, carefully, as she signed her name in loopy letters, far bigger than they used to be. I remember how sad it was each time for me to see just her name, solo and without my grandfather's beside it. But the sadness passed as with each card came a memory, a story. I listened intently, wanting to remember every detail, as she reminisced about family back in England and dear friends who had been there for her for fifty years or more.

I sent each card away and it wasn't until years later that I found out just how much it meant to the people who received them that we had taken the time to do this.

HEATHER, MISSISSAUGA, ONTARIO

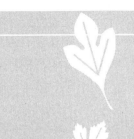
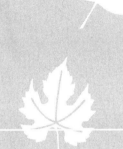

4

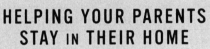

HELPING YOUR PARENTS
STAY in THEIR HOME

As your parents enter their middle senior years and experience the natural physical changes of aging they may find their house more than they can cope with. Yet many older people want to stay in their home for as long as possible. With all the changes happening at this stage of their lives, their home provides a haven of familiarity and stability, and also contributes a great deal to their sense of personal independence. At this point you and your parents together will need to determine what changes may have to be put in place so that they can stay in their home safely and securely. In this chapter we explore

- how aging and physical change impacts safety in the home
- the importance of preventing falls
- touring your parents' home for hazards
- how to modify the home for easy living and safety
- assistive devices
- arranging informal and formal home care
- social services care workers and what they do for your parents
- questions to ask about in-home care providers.

How Aging Impacts Safety in the Home

If your parents are to be able to stay at home, they will require two key elements: a safe home environment and caregiver support. It is imperative that you observe your parents' daily activities and identify areas that are becoming difficult for them to manage. Your parents will rely on you to help them to adapt so that they can take care of the house and themselves.

Recognizing the Physical Changes

As we age our senses become less sharp and this can lead to accidents in the home. Be aware that your parents' vision, hearing, touch, smell, mobility, reaction time, balance and memory will all become less sensitive. Stretching, lifting and bending become more difficult, so accessibility is crucial. Be proactive! Making adjustments to the house in anticipation of these changes will make it easier for your parents to enjoy their surroundings safely.

HOW AGING DIMINISHES THE SENSES

- Vision: it takes longer to adjust to light from dark areas.
- Depth perception: it's more difficult to judge distances, for example walking down the stairs.
- Touch: it's harder to detect pain and know when things are hot or cold.
- Hearing loss: it's difficult to hear phones and alarms.
- Mobility, balance and reaction times: it takes longer to get things done and is harder to get around.
- Memory: it's easy to forget to turn off the stove or take medications.
- Cognitive function: it becomes difficult to make decisions and think through a problem logically.

The Danger of Falls in the Home

One of the most important things you can do is to put in place safety measures to prevent falls in the home. If our parents fall, it takes a long time for them to heal and the injuries can lead to further complications. As well, a fall can make a senior fearful and hesitant to continue in their normal routine.

Falls account for more than half the injuries among Canadians aged sixty-five years and older. The likelihood of dying from a fall-related injury increases with age. Among seniors, 20 percent of deaths related to injury can be traced back to a fall. Falls are the leading cause of injury-related admissions, accounting for 79 percent of seniors' hospitalizations.[11]

A fall or even a decline in the senses can make your parents feel inadequate and not capable of doing things for themselves. It is our responsibility as caregivers to help establish an environment where our parents can concentrate on what they can do rather than what they can't, allowing them to maintain their sense of achievement and autonomy.

Pay attention to tasks your parents are having difficulty completing. During regular visits, observe your parents and communicate with them. Making modifications to their home will allow your parents to remain in their home longer and more safely.

Touring the Home for Hazards

The first thing to do is to assess the home and see what improvements need to be made. Touring the home with your parents is an opportunity for them to point out areas where they are having difficulties.

This could be an eye-opener for you as a caregiver. You may not have been aware of the problems your parents are having. When you tour the home you will be surprised at some of the simple modifications that can be made, such as removing rugs

Our house is shared with two big dogs—dogs with toys, bones and balls. I became conscious of how often their stuff was left scattered around the house: bones at the top of the stairs; stuffed toys in the middle of the hallway; and balls in bedroom doorways. They're just like kids, except I can't make them responsible for picking up after themselves, so I became compulsive about moving things out of the walkways and putting things into baskets scattered around the house.

I never noticed how much stuff lay scattered about until my mom developed cataracts and had trouble seeing. Then I worried about her tripping and falling. A couple of times I had to call out "Mom, look down" as she almost stepped in the dog's dish that had been nosed into the middle of the floor.

My mom almost had a spill on the stairs when the dogs were younger so we trained them to go up and down the stairs on one side leaving the handrail free for whoever is on the stairs with them.

I think the hardest thing was to remember that how I moved around, and what I saw was not what my mom was experiencing. She wasn't as mobile as me, didn't react as quickly as me and didn't see what I saw, especially at night.

LINDA

from main traffic areas and using nightlights in the hallways. If your parents require more physical assistance, however, you will need to consider more extensive modifications, such as installing grab bars in the bathtub or renovating the front entrance for a ramp. These changes can make a world of difference in your parents' daily lives.

HOME SAFETY: TOURING THE HOME CHECKLIST[12]

Does the outside entrance have

- [ ] properly positioned outdoor lighting fixtures with bulb wattage high enough to light the walkway and the house number?
- [ ] a house number in a visible location (day or night)?
- [ ] railings on exterior stairs?
- [ ] stairs in good condition and free of clutter?
- [ ] a mailbox that is visible and easy to access?

Generally throughout the home is/are there

- [ ] lighting in hallways that is bright enough for your parents?
- [ ] throw rugs secured in place to prevent tripping?
- [ ] high traffic areas clear of clutter and obstacles?
- [ ] pets out from underfoot?
- [ ] seating at doorways to remove and put on shoes?
- [ ] first aid kits easily accessible on all floors of the house?
- [ ] lists of emergency phone numbers near all phones in the house?
- [ ] doors with lever handles that allow for easy opening?

Are the stairs

- [ ] sufficiently lit top to bottom?
- [ ] equipped with light switches at the top and bottom?
- [ ] free of throw rugs to prevent tripping?
- [ ] free of clutter and obstacles?
- [ ] outfitted with a non-skid surface?
- [ ] equipped with sturdy handrails at a height of 36 inches to 39 inches?

To prevent fire

- [ ] are there smoke detectors on every floor of the home and are they tested every six months?
- [ ] is there a planned escape route?
- [ ] is there a carbon monoxide alarm in the home?
- [ ] are flammable and hazardous materials clearly labelled and properly stored?
- [ ] are space heaters placed well away from flammable substances and materials?
- [ ] are power bars being used to prevent overloading electrical outlets?
- [ ] has an electrician inspected the wiring and fuse box if you have an older home?
- [ ] are electrical cords in good condition and secured away from walkways?
- [ ] are small appliances in good condition?
- [ ] are there appropriate fire extinguishers throughout the home?

Does the bathroom have

- [ ] the hot water temperature set to the recommended 49°C (120°F)?
- [ ] non-slip surfaces in the tub or shower?
- [ ] bath mats with rubberized backing at the tub or shower to prevent slipping?
- [ ] a night-light?
- [ ] a door lock with an exterior emergency release?
- [ ] grab bars in the tub, shower and toilet that are properly placed and well anchored?
- [ ] a shower with a hand-held shower head?
- [ ] sink faucets with easy-lever handles?

Does the kitchen have

- ☐ frequently used cooking equipment and foods stored in easy-to-reach locations, ideally between knee and shoulder height?
- ☐ heavy items stored in the lower cupboards and lighter items in the higher cupboards?
- ☐ a stable stepstool with a safety rail for reaching high places?
- ☐ a stove with clearly marked "on" and "off" dials?
- ☐ a fire extinguisher mounted on the wall away from the stove?
- ☐ small appliances with automatic shutoffs?
- ☐ appliances and equipment with easy-to-read and easy-to-reach dials?
- ☐ utensils with large handles for easy gripping?
- ☐ reachers to help get objects or food?
- ☐ pot stabilizers to prevent the pot from moving while stirring or pot watchers to prevent boiling over?

Does the bedroom have

- ☐ a light switch near the entrance?
- ☐ lamps or a light switch near the bed?
- ☐ a bed at a height that your parents can get in and out of easily?
- ☐ night-lights for visibility in the middle of the night?
- ☐ a clear path from the bed to the bathroom?
- ☐ a phone and a list of emergency phone numbers near the bed?
- ☐ floors that are clear of clutter and obstacles?

Does the garage/basement/laundry room have

- ☐ sufficient lighting in the work area?
- ☐ an accessible telephone and a list of emergency phone numbers?

- [ ] floors that are clear of clutter to prevent tripping?
- [ ] tools and service equipment that are in good working order?
- [ ] equipment that's stored securely with working safety locks?
- [ ] well-ventilated work areas for both summer and winter?
- [ ] shelves or cupboards that allow heavy items to be stored on lower levels for easy access?
- [ ] a ladder or a stable stepstool (with a safety rail) for reaching high places?
- [ ] chemicals, such as bleach, cleaners and paint thinners clearly identified?
- [ ] proper storage for flammable materials as indicated on the labels, away from sources of heat and flame?

PERSONAL SAFETY TIPS

- Remind your parents to remove their reading glasses when going up and down the stairs.
- When your parents rise from sitting or lying down, suggest they pause before walking. This will prevent them from fainting due to low blood pressure.
- Encourage them not to hurry, and especially to take their time on the stairs.
- Make sure they are registered on their apartment building's fire safety plan if they need assistance exiting the building in an emergency.
- Remind your parents to test the water temperature before getting into the bath or shower.
- Remind your parents never to cook while wearing loose-fitting clothing or sleepwear.

If your parents have special needs or you are not able to tour the home with them, contact seniors organizations for help in assessing their house. Check with your home insurance company to see what is covered under your plan should major modifications be required. The Canada Mortgage and Housing Corporation offers financial assistance for home renovations based on financial eligibility. (See our Senior and Caregiver Resource Guide for contact information.)

Environmental gerontologist: an interior designer with expertise in modifying residences to accommodate the stages of aging without too much of a change to the house's aesthetic. This is a relatively new field that is destined to grow as the population ages.

Assistive Devices

By using assistive devices, your parents can prevent injuries and remain physically and mentally active. Such devices can make the difference between something being easy to do and something being difficult and frustrating, or even dangerous. You may find, however, that your parents are resistant to them because they think they make them look or feel old. Keeping your goal of personal dignity in mind, you will need to approach this subject with sensitivity. Once convinced, your parents may find the value of these devices far outweighs the negatives.

Some of these devices can be rented or purchased through your local drugstore or medical supplier. In some cases, you may be required to make arrangements through your family doctor. Check your provincial health care plan or your private health care insurance carrier to see if any of these are covered.

If your parents have trouble walking, canes and appropriate footwear can help. Or in more serious cases, consider getting them a walker. Some even have seats to rest on. If they have

My father was leaving the hospital and needed to get a walking aid quickly. He had a rental wheelchair and now was graduating to a cane or walker. We tried the cane but it did not give enough support and several times he actually tripped on it. I turned to the walker after several people suggested it would be the most useful. I did a quick search on the Internet to get approximate prices, things to look for and styles. In the store the staff was very helpful, asking many questions that I hadn't even thought about. I couldn't take him with me, which would have been much more helpful in purchasing the correct size. The questions they had were what is his height and weight? Will he want to carry things with him? Will it be for indoor or outdoor walking? Will it need brakes? What type of seat did he want? I had to remind myself that I was buying a walker not a car, but I was glad they pointed out these options to me.

A walker that is the correct height encourages him to walk upright and helps prevent him from hunching over it. I also discovered that a comfortable seat is important because he uses it all the time. Standing for long periods of time is not an option. I'm glad I got brakes on the walker because I'm sure without them we could be back to using a wheelchair. I purchased a very lightweight walker because lifting it in and out of the car is trying. Also make sure that it fits in your car. Nothing is more frustrating than a walker that is a few inches too big for the trunk. When he downsized his room, we were glad to see that the walker still fit through the bathroom door and around the bed. Most falls take place within a senior's own rooms, so using his walker all the time helps prevent a fall. I'm glad my father was willing to use a walker because without it I'm sure we would be in a different situation today.

CAREGIVER, TORONTO, ONTARIO

trouble seeing, find large-pad touch-tone phones, and arrange magnifying glasses strategically around the house near phones, reading chairs and bill-paying areas. If your parents have trouble hearing, they can check with their doctor about hearing aid options. You can look into getting a telephone with volume controls, and flashing lights for the doorbell. Encourage the use of memory aids, especially with medication; have your parents write down information, keep a pad and pencil by the phone, put pictures on cupboards, and use a pill organizer and/or a timer to help them remember to take their medication.

Consider purchasing an emergency response system for your parents. These usually involve your parents wearing a band on their arm or a pendant around their neck; on it is a button that they can push to alert the company if they need help. Like a burglary alarm company, these companies request a priority list of people to contact in case of an emergency. In the event that family cannot be reached, the company dispatches emergency support. This service is especially useful and can give you peace of mind if your parents live far from you.

In-Home Care: A Support System

There may come a time when you need to arrange outside help for your parents. Their care needs can change overnight, and you need to be alert to this possibility. Often the additional help required is due to a decline in your parents' health. Or perhaps your

 Convincing my mother to use aids was difficult. Rather than get upset with her I always used humour, because she had a wonderful sense of humour. Her cane wasn't used for walking, it was a dog-shooing stick, and for the diapers I asked her if I could borrow one as I had a cold and would keep peeing myself every time I coughed. She laughed and began wearing them.

I will never get my mother back but I know I did everything I could for her at the time.

KIM, MAPLE RIDGE,
BRITISH COLUMBIA

HELPING YOUR PARENTS STAY IN THEIR HOME

own situation has changed and the amount of help you can provide is less than what's required due to the responsibility of a full-time job, family obligations or distance from your parents' home.

Perhaps your parents are starting to require personal or medical care that you do not have the experience to give, or they aren't comfortable with you, their adult child, helping them, especially with personal needs.

There are several different types of care available. The key is to remember that you are putting in place a support system to allow your parents to be as independent as possible for as long as possible.

DEFINING FORMAL AND INFORMAL CARE

Formal care describes care provided by professionals, whether in a home environment or in a retirement home, hospital or long-term care facility. *Informal care* describes care provided by family members, friends and volunteers.

Informal Care Options

Your parents may already be receiving casual help through family, friends or neighbours. This assistance can be invaluable and should not be overlooked as a significant part of your parents' care. As they require increasing levels of care, however, you will need to set up a more structured support system. Before moving to formal care options, have a conversation with your parents about their routines to figure out what support they already have in place.

Perhaps neighbours and family are keeping a casual eye on your parents' coming and goings, or are dropping by to help around the house or driving them to appointments. This sporadic support will need to become more formal, so that you can keep an eye on your parents' progress and know when additional care is needed. For example, a neighbour may agree to always take the garbage to the curb on garbage day and your sister will be responsible to drive your mom to a weekly appointment and both will contact you if they become concerned about your parents. Your parents will feel less isolated if they know that people are coming by to check in on them. But be careful not to overburden friends and neighbours.

Having other people help also gives you as the caregiver an opportunity for a break. Allow other people to take on some responsibilities. You may even decide to have your parents alternate long-term visits among siblings. Don't be afraid to ask for help, and to accept it!

Formal Care Options in the Home

To help you determine the level of outside care your parents need, consider their daily activities, how comfortable you are providing care in problem areas, how accessible you are and how the care will fit into your schedule, and their medical requirements. You can make arrangements with personal care services or homemaking services or both.

Personal care services deal with your parents' physical needs and are often based on medical and mobility issues. *Homemaking services* assist with the house maintenance and transportation.

Personal care and homemaking services can be arranged through a variety of providers: government agencies, support groups, community services, nursing care agencies, retail services and volunteers. Unfortunately, putting this formal care in place does not necessarily reduce the amount of assistance you are providing. In fact, you will have to supervise the formal care providers to make sure they are doing what's necessary, and to your parents' satisfaction.

Social services agencies can assist you in determining what types of care are available to your parents. In each province a specialized government agency will assign a case manager or coordinator (usually a social worker or registered nurse) to assess your parents' care needs and eligibility and work with your parents to develop a care plan. This person will also

- stay in touch with you in case of any change in care needs, reassessing at regular intervals

WHAT DO PERSONAL CARE AND HOMEMAKING SERVICES PROVIDE?

Personal care providers

- administer medication and change wound dressings
- assist with personal hygiene, dressing and bathing
- help your parents eat
- assist with transfers (for example, moving from a bed to a wheelchair).

Homemaking services provide

- light housekeeping
- meal planning
- meal delivery
- shopping
- laundry
- bill payment
- transportation.

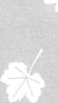

Formal care providers include

- social workers
- home support workers
- occupational therapists
- physiotherapists
- registered nurses (RN), registered practical nurses (RPN) and licensed practical nurses (LPN)
- homemaking services
- adult day programs.

- offer a link to support services available to seniors and help to coordinate them
- determine if your parents can stay in their home safely and give suggestions on how to modify the home
- provide information on housing options such as remaining at home
- coordinate and interview for in-home support services, supportive housing and long-term care facilities
- determine eligibility for services and funding
- become an advocate for your parents in trying to arrange services.

See our Senior and Caregiver Resource Guide under Social Services Support and Assessment for contact information for the agency in your province.

Working with Your Parents to Put Help in Place

This time—during which you and your parents adjust to having outside help come into the home—can be difficult and stressful. Consider your parents' preferences throughout this process. Perhaps they would like to have some formal care and some informal care, depending on the activity. Your mom may prefer it if you help her take a bath, but your dad may prefer these personal tasks be done through formal care.

You may find it harder than you expect to trust other people to take care of your parents. There will be a difficult adjustment period until you *and* your parents get used to having someone else intimately involved in the caregiving.

> When my grandmother had congestive heart failure we soon realized we weren't up for the daily needles. Whenever she answered the door and recognized her home care worker she would be thrilled because it meant she wouldn't be jabbed by her inexperienced family members.
>
> KENDALL, TORONTO, ONTARIO

Your parents may resist the idea of having strangers come into the house. It's important to acknowledge and respect their feelings. You will need to have an open and honest conversation about how much care you are able to provide. Offer to be with them for the first few visits with the formal care provider for their comfort and security. Be realistic with them so that they recognize your limitations as a caregiver. Through this conversation they should realize that additional formal care will help them to live more productive and active lives in their home.

If their resistance continues after your conversations, your social services case manager may be able to intervene with your parents and work with them to find out why they are unwilling to accept help. If they continue to refuse your help and are still capable of making their own choices, you will have to come to

My sister and I lived hours away, which left my brother to tend to our parents as best he could, while coping with his own serious health issues, [or] more aptly, as much as they would let him on a day-to-day basis. Theirs was a classic case of self-neglect. We could all see the signs. We all tried to reason with both of them to accept home care, which was available to them. We offered a variety of supports designed to keep them safe and comfortable in their own home for as long as possible. These efforts were met with abject refusal. Children didn't tell their parents how to live their lives. In their minds, they were absolutely fine and didn't need anything. Because my mother would not allow any professionals into the home, they couldn't be assessed properly. They wouldn't even visit the doctor. When asked, they said everything was just fine. Legally, their right to autonomy precluded any direct intervention. Their health deteriorated, but no amount of persuasion from their children or anyone else could get through to them.

LESLEY, TORONTO, ONTARIO

terms with this, knowing that you have done all you can to offer assistance.

The Questions You Should Ask

It may be time-consuming to try to arrange the resources they need, but once these are in place you'll be relieved to know that your parents are getting the best support possible. Knowing what questions to ask when setting up formal care will give you confidence in the provider coming into the home.

If you are paying privately, you can find formal care providers through your yellow pages or online under "home health services," "nurses" or "homemaker services." You may even consider a live-in arrangement with the care provider.

QUESTIONS TO ASK ABOUT YOUR CARE PROVIDER

Ability to Provide Care for Your Parents

- Does the formal care provider have the services to be able to meet your parents' needs?
- Do they have specific requirements (level of care, financial need, service area) that your parents' have to meet?
- What is their application process?
- Do they have waiting times and how long are these?
- Is there a cost for the service and are there standard fees? How are costs calculated? How will you be billed?
- Are your parents eligible for fee subsidies through the provincial/ federal governments or their private insurance plan?
- What types of services are available?
- What specifically will be provided within the service?

Qualifications of the Formal Care Provider

- Can the provider supply references for their staff?
- Is there a contract outlining responsibilities for both the care provider and your parents?
- Are the staff specially trained? And what types of staff and volunteers provide the service?
- Does the same person come regularly? And if not, how do you know who is coming?
- Can you interview the staff/volunteers who will come into the home?
- Who supervises the staff/volunteers and how can you contact them?

- Who will be your contact for general information and/or to modify care arrangements?
- Is the provider approved by a provincial association or other accrediting body—for example, Canadian Council on Health Services Accreditation (CCHSA) or International Organization for Standardization (ISO 9001)?
- Are they a member of an association, such as a registered massage therapist, the chiropractic association, or a registered physiotherapist?
- Do they have precautions to ensure your security? For example, are volunteers/staff bonded, have background checks been done, have qualifications been confirmed?
- Do they have liability insurance?
- What is their complaint process?
- What are the limitations of the service? For example, the days/hours of operation, what is not provided?

Adapted from Ministry of Health and Long-Term Care Ontario, "Home & Community Services Checklist."

There may come a time, however, when staying at home is no longer an option. In the next chapter we look at alternative living arrangements.

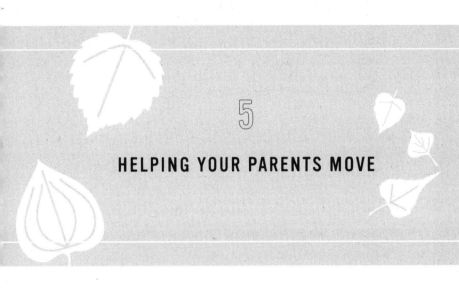

5

HELPING YOUR PARENTS MOVE

We now turn our attention to what happens when it is time for your parents to move out of their home, and how you can help them to decide where to live. We will look at

- why your parents are moving
- the impact and financial considerations of selling the family home
- condominiums, apartments, life-lease housing, retirement residences and supportive housing
- families moving in together
- assisted living facilities and long-term care homes
- staying home for the duration of care.

Deciding to Move

One of the most visible and significant changes for you and your parents comes when they realize that it's time to sell their house. No matter what the reason for moving, giving up the home will be a sad time for the family.

There are many different reasons that your parents may make the difficult decision to move: the house is too big and hard to maintain, they want access to the equity, they lead an active lifestyle and don't want the responsibility of a house, they can no

Grandma Jean is a wonderful lady, very loving, caring and the best grandma anyone could ask for. A few years ago, while she was living on her own, she fell and broke a hip while standing on a chair, changing a fuse in the top of her stove. Her life went downhill from there. We had a family meeting with her doctor and it was decided that Grandma had to go to a retirement home or possibly a nursing home. We did our homework and looked for the perfect home, offering the right amount of care, while making her feel she wasn't losing her independence. We ended up choosing a place that offered a "lodge" as well as a nursing home floor.

The best time to visit is when there is a program on. You go and attend the program with them, and it gets them out of their room, spending time doing something together, while you have a visit with them. Then you take them back to their room while they are happy and discuss how enjoyable it was and look at their monthly calendar to decide when you can come back to do that again. Doing this eliminates a great deal of the stress, for both of you.

Working in a nursing home you see everything and it makes you more aware of what signs to look for when you have one of your parents in one. Their appearance, the attitude of the staff, and the cleanliness of the building are just a few of the things to look for. Visit during mealtime; offer to help feed a resident who isn't capable of feeding themselves so you can observe the surroundings and the atmosphere in the dining rooms. Working in a nursing home can be very busy and very demanding, but no resident should be hurried through their meal. Look for these signs and if you see something you don't like, tell the director of resident care. They need to know. Your parent might be able to tell you if they don't like something, but there are residents that can't talk and they can't say what is wrong so you need to be their voice.

Visits from family and friends are the most important thing elderly people have to look forward to, so visit as often as possible and bring those little ones with you, and if you see a piano or an organ and you are talented enough to play a song or two, please play for them. They love it! The smiles on their faces are amazing. Watching them tap their feet or clap their hands to the music sure makes my day.

Being in a nursing home isn't what we truly want for our loved ones, but there are excellent homes out there and the key to finding the right home is to go there, spend time, and talk with the residents. Ask the cleaning lady which residents you should talk to, she will know. For me, working in a nursing home is the most rewarding job out there. I feel very lucky to have all those grandmas and grandpas. I love them all!

LISA, ST. MARY'S, ONTARIO

longer afford to live in their home, they need increasing care or are anticipating future care needs, or one of your parents is widowed and cannot maintain the house. A sudden decline in one or both parents' health or a medical crisis may be the determining factor.

Often aging parents are in denial about their situation and it will be up to you to suggest that it's time to move. A key factor affecting this decision is your parents' health and the degree to which they are able to remain independent. Similarly, the amount of care your parents will require is going to determine their new living arrangements. You will need to discuss with your parents what accommodations would best suit their lifestyle and whether they already have plans in place. No matter what the reasons for the move, a number of factors come into play: finances, care needs, and proximity to family members, amenities, transportation, shopping, community and friends. These factors may conflict with one another, so it's important to weigh them and determine which should take precedence. For example, it may be more important at this stage that they be close to you than that they stay in their own neighbourhood.

When choosing a new home for your parents, try to think long term to reduce the number of changes your parents must endure. For example, if your parents are downsizing to a condominium, look for one close to a long-term facility so they are already familiar with the neighbourhood.

Moving is a major life change and no matter what the reason your parents are considering making a move, it should be well thought out and not made in haste. For example, the passing of your father does not necessarily mean your mother must immediately move out of her home.

Selling the Family Home

Once your parents have decided to move, they will have to make plans to sell their house if they own it. Support your parents as they adjust to this major change in their lives. Their home is connected to feelings of accomplishment and independence. There may be considerable work involved in preparing your parents' house for sale in order to get the best selling price. Your real estate agent or an independent appraiser can give you suggestions on improvements that can increase the value of the home.

My parents' home was always the gathering place for my large family. Everyone knew that special occasions were celebrated there and there was always an open invitation to drop by. I knew whenever I visited I'd likely find someone else there when I arrived. Now that my parents have moved, it takes a bit more effort to figure out whose house everyone is going to meet at for the next event. But the heart of the family is still there even if the address is different, and I realize now that's more important.

BARBARA

Selling your parents' home often elicits many opinions from everyone in the family. This is an emotional decision as well as a practical one, and each person may have a different idea of what course of action is best. It's especially difficult if all family members don't agree that there *is* a need to sell the home. There may be conflict. Everyone should keep in mind that you're all trying to do the best thing for your parents in the long term.

Factors that Have an Impact on Moving

As your parents age, their financial circumstances will affect what future living options you consider. Long-term financial planning is important to take into account. Perhaps your parents have already organized their finances for their senior years and it's a simple matter of putting their plans in place. But it's also possible that your parents have not saved enough to cover their future needs and that you will need to sit down to realistically assess what housing options and living expenses they can afford. Though the least expensive option is sometimes staying in their own home, this is not always possible. You and your siblings may even have to contribute financially to help your parents make the appropriate move. If your parents' finances are complicated, consult a financial adviser.

Once you've determined what they can afford, help your parents investigate the options. They may know of some facilities that have been recommended by friends. Accompany them to tour these places. It's helpful to take with you a checklist of things that your parents would like to have in their new home, and think about questions they should ask, for example details of the rental agreement. Take a ride around the neighbourhood to see how easy it is to get to places of importance such as the grocery store, pharmacy, religious centre, community centre, doctors' offices, and, of course, your home and those of other family members.

I helped pack up my parents' house that they had lived in for over forty years. There were many rooms to sift through and many memories recalled in the process. On the closing day, some of my family met up for one last dinner at the house. Since the house was empty we all found spots to sit on the floor and kitchen counter. Our voices echoed through the house as we talked about the good times we had shared in our home.

Before leaving I took a walk through each room by myself just to have one last look at the place where I grew up. Even the garage had my sisters' and brothers' chalk writing on the walls. It was strange to lock the door for one last time knowing we would not be going in the house again. I looked back before leaving and tried to stamp all the details in my mind: the beautiful garden that my mom was so proud of, the house number above the garage and the image that I knew as home. It was a good way to say goodbye to a wonderful home as it helped me find peace with the decision. I have not been back, as I don't want that image in my mind to disappear. And I can turn my attention to a new phase in my parents' lives and my own as I help them to create new memories in their new homes.

BARBARA

Based on your parents' level of independence and their care requirements, there are a variety of living options available.

Condominiums and Apartments

Condominiums and apartments give your parents their own space but relieve them of the responsibilities of a house. These facilities also may have amenities such as pools or exercise rooms.

If your parents are moving from a house to an apartment, this will be an adjustment. Have a conversation with them in the planning stages about the differences between the environments. In an apartment they may hear more noise from neighbours and in the hallways, they may smell cooking odours, and they will have to deal with condo associations and landlords. If one of your parents has lost his or her partner and is not used to living without familiar neighbours nearby, he or she may find it difficult to adapt to the solitary surroundings. As a caregiver you need to be aware that seniors are at risk for depression and feelings of isolation, so an apartment environment may not be suitable. Look at all your parents' options and bear in mind their personalities when deciding whether downsizing to an apartment or condominium is the right choice.

Life-Lease Housing

Life-lease housing is a unique living option that is becoming increasingly popular among seniors. They are modelled after condominium projects and have similar suite options, features and monthly fees, and similar management, maintenance, insurance and a building reserve fund. However, the owner on title is a not-for-profit or charitable organization. Your parents can purchase a life-lease interest, at market value, in both the property and their suite. They have exclusive use of the suite and shared use of common areas and facilities. Some facilities provide support services for your parents' changing care needs. This lease interest can pass on to the family upon your parents' death. In some provinces, if your parents decide to sell their interest, they will receive market value. The non-profit corporation must approve the sale or transfer.

Unlike condominiums there is an age restriction for residents. Some seniors are choosing life-lease housing because they offer a sense of community and access to a variety of services. This type of housing option is not available in all the provinces and regulations vary. Search online for life-lease housing in your province for more information.

Retirement Residences

Retirement residences, another option for independent living, allow your parents to live in an apartment and at the same time socialize with people of similar ages and with similar interests. Retirement residences are privately owned rental housing and as a result they are not government subsidized and can range in price significantly. They are also not regulated by the government, so it's critical that you ask questions and pay close attention when previewing them. Be an alert consumer on your parents' behalf. Retirement residences commonly offer packages that include meals and services. They can provide some support and care while allowing seniors to live independently with access to social activities and amenities.

Retirement residences usually offer a range of room sizes, good security (because there are others living close by), and are ideal for individuals who still have active lifestyles and don't need a high level of care. Some offer graduated levels of care, which may be important in helping your parents adapt to future personal care and health needs.

Retirement homes also can be affiliated with cultural or religious communities, something to consider if your parents find it easier to communicate and relate with people who have similar backgrounds and traditions. In other cases the cultural makeup of the facility may be a reflection of its location.

Retirement homes are often very social places with a main dining room, lounge areas and planned activities. This can be beneficial if your parents enjoy others' company. On the other hand, your parents may not think of themselves as old and may not want to socialize only with people their own age and older. But before rejecting the idea of a retirement home, visit one with your parents so they can see what it's like. If they would like to consider a retirement home as an option, preview a couple of residences to compare their features and get a good idea of what is available.

PREVIEWING RETIREMENT RESIDENCES CHECKLIST

Financial and Administrative

☐ What room layouts are available?

☐ How much does it cost monthly/annually?

☐ What are the terms of the lease agreement?

☐ How often do rates increase? And what is the annual rate of increase over the last few years?

☐ What is the application process?

☐ Are the employees bonded?

☐ Is there a waiting list and/or what is available and in what time frame?

☐ Are there visitor restrictions?

☐ What are the security features? Is there an assistive alarm system in place?

☐ How much notice do you need to give if you decide to move out?

☐ Does the facility have affiliations with a specific ethnic or religious community?

Health Care

☐ Is a health assessment required?

☐ Is there wheelchair accessibility?

☐ What happens if your parents' health deteriorates?

☐ Can the facility adapt to the changing needs of your parents? What type of personal care does it offer? Is there a charge for extra services?

- [ ] Are there higher levels of care available if needed in the future?
- [ ] Will the home assist your parents when they need to apply for higher levels of care?
- [ ] How close is the nearest hospital? What are the emergency/fire procedures?

Services and Amenities

- [ ] What optional services are available and at what cost?
- [ ] Is phone and cable included in the cost?
- [ ] What are some sample menus? Do they have choices?
- [ ] What services are provided (laundry, housekeeping, recreational activities)?
- [ ] Is there parking available?
- [ ] Are there transportation options?
- [ ] Is there a private meeting/dining area to entertain family or friends? Is a kitchen available to use?

Even after your parents have made the move to a retirement residence you will still have responsibilities as their caregiver. In the majority of cases, the residence is not responsible for monitoring your parents' changing health care needs. Remain vigilant and stay involved and aware of your parents' progress and keep the lines of communication open. It's also important for other family members to visit often and communicate with you in your role as caregiver.

Supportive Housing

Supportive housing offers affordable accommodations to seniors who require varying levels of care and support but don't require twenty-four-hour medical attention. Assistance such as meals, housekeeping, transportation, twenty-four-hour emergency response, some personal care needs, social activities and daily visits are available. Accommodations can range in style and layout; some can be apartment-style dwellings while others can be shared rooms. They often have common amenities, such as activity rooms, dining rooms and lounges. This type of housing can be rented or owned like a condo or a life-lease, or it can be non-profit or for-profit with costs that vary depending on ownership. Some facilities are partially funded by the government. For both government-funded and private facilities, your parents may need to meet eligibility requirements based on age, income and care needs. Your provincial social service agency can help you to determine eligibility and assist with applications for provincially funded facilities.

Moving in with the Kids

For some people the decision to have their parents move in with them is easily made. Others struggle to come to terms with their parents sharing their home. It doesn't matter how independent your parents are, if they live with you your involvement will be 24/7, so this decision will have an impact on all aspects of your life. It will affect your social activities, your holiday plans, your work; it can cause changes in sleep patterns due to stress or new demands on your time; it can stretch your finances; it can affect your health. This new dynamic will also require changes to all the family roles. In making the decision as to whether your parents should live with you, you need to be honest and not let guilt pressure you into taking on more than you can handle. You also need to take into account your own health and abilities, and your comfort level in providing personal care for your aging parents.

Depending on your family structure, it may be obvious who is able to offer this option to your parents. In some cases, however, especially with a large family, it may be less clear. Or this role may automatically fall on you as the caregiver. Have an honest discussion with your immediate family. Talk over all the possibilities with them and tell them what your parents will require and how their presence in your home will affect their daily routine. It's important to understand and take into consideration

> At the time of her diagnosis it was obvious my mother couldn't live on her own, so I invited her to move in with my family, without even discussing it with my husband. We lived in a small house with our thirteen-year-old daughter. [My mother] moved in, and I became her full-time caregiver. When she first moved in she was unable to swallow and eventually her speech and walking disappeared. She also suffered from dementia. I became the parent. . . . My daughter had to move out of her room because it was the biggest. My mother was finally fitted with a feeding tube in her stomach, which made it easier for me. She could not be left alone, which meant we could never go out as a family; someone had to be with her to feed her.
>
> I tried not to treat her like a child and still think of her as my mother, but each day brought new challenges. Trying to keep her mind active was difficult for me because of the lack of sleep and responsibilities that went along with caring for an elderly parent.
>
> KIM, MAPLE RIDGE, BRITISH COLUMBIA

their feelings as this is going to have an impact on their lives too. Make sure everyone in the family gets a chance to voice their concerns regarding privacy issues, schedules, finances and bills. Think carefully about the dynamics between your parents and other family members and decide whether the move is a realistic one for all concerned.

Your family will also need to be aware of the physical changes that come with aging such as forgetfulness and loss of hearing, and they must learn to have patience and empathy. You may have to change how your household functions and establish practices around such things as clutter and lighting. Whether it's a choice, or the only option, everyone in the family will need to adapt.

Evaluate Your Own Home

If you decide to invite your parents to move in with you, evaluate your home to see how it suits their needs, now and for the future. Is your house set up to provide proper care for your parents and a comfortable place for them to live? Do you need to renovate to create a private area for your parents? Do they have mobility issues? Is it necessary to keep them on the main level? Is there a washroom accessible? Also, do you need to accommodate a walker or wheelchair? If renovations aren't enough, you may even have to think about selling your current home to buy a new one that will suit everyone's needs.

When your parents move in, their daily activities will need to be incorporated into your household routine. Immediate family members will need to help out, so let them know what is expected of them. Extended family too should be involved. Just because your parents have moved in with you doesn't mean your siblings or other family are no longer responsible. For example, they might take your mom or dad out for a couple of hours on a regular basis so that you can have some time for yourself.

Don't try to do everything on your own; ask others to help. Recognizing the changes in everyone's life as a result of this move is very important.

Don't forget that your parents will be emotional during this time as well. They may feel that they are becoming a burden to you and interfering in your life. Let them know that you feel this

One afternoon, my mom, my son and I were sitting having lunch. My mom was complaining about some aches and pains: "I'm getting old."

My three-year-old son looked over and said, "We need a new Gramma."

"Where would we get a new Gramma from?" I replied.

"From the grocery store in aisle G."

My mom and I started laughing.

Then he said, "No, we don't need a new Gramma. You're my best friend."

After fifty-eight happy years of marriage, nine kids and living in the same house for forty-nine years, my mom came to live with us about a year and a half ago. My dad moved into a retirement home, which offered nursing care. He has been diagnosed with Alzheimer's disease. It has been very difficult for my mom. She has never lived on her own or been away from my dad. My husband and I knew that she needed to be somewhere with family.

It is wonderful to see smiles on her face again and hear the laughter in her voice when she spends time with her grandson. And somehow that makes it a little easier. Now, I often hear reverberating throughout the house, "Come on Gramma, let's go play," and that brings a smile to my face too.

BERNADETTE, OAKVILLE, ONTARIO

THINGS TO CONSIDER BEFORE PARENTS MOVE IN

- What are your parents' wishes?
- Are the relationships between your parents and the extended family members (son-in-laws, daughter-in-laws and grandchildren) conducive to living together?
- How do all members of the family feel about it?
- What are your parents' care requirements and are you able to provide for them now or in the future (personally or with formal care)?
- Is the arrangement going to be permanent or temporary? Does everyone in the family understand how long it may continue?
- Are there other circumstances within your immediate family that will influence the decision? For example, health issues or work schedules.
- How will you maintain one another's personal space and privacy?
- Does the house layout let your parents have their own accommodation?
- Can the house be modified to suit the family's needs?
- What are the financial ramifications for your parents and your family, and extended family?

is a positive change for you and your family. If you have children, a strong relationship can develop between grandchildren and grandparents that helps the young ones develop respect for seniors and create wonderful memories that will last a lifetime.

It can also be stressful for your spouse as your family adjusts to the new living arrangement. You may find yourself acting as a mediator between your spouse and parents as you try to take everyone's feelings into account. If everyone involved admits

My mom moved to the same city that I live in two years ago. It was so great to finally have her in the same town as me, as I would not have to worry about her as much and could care for her. They were many things to do to get her settled in her new home, and one of them was finding a Catholic Church for her to attend. I had been Anglican for a number of years, but not attending, although very strong in my faith. I mentioned to my mom that it would be great if we could both find and go to an Anglican Church, which did not go over very well.

So I did find a Catholic Church, and we both started attending. I suddenly remembered all the times when as a child, my mom had reached out and put my hand in hers and the safety and love I felt, and now she was receiving this gift from me. The tears rolled down my cheeks as I squeezed her hand and thought now it is my turn to look after her. Needless to say, we attend the Catholic Church every Sunday together.

CAREGIVER, KITCHENER, ONTARIO

how difficult the situation is and makes an effort to get along, then there can be benefits for all. Your parents will feel cared for by you, and they will also be active and involved in family, making them feel productive and useful.

Making the Move Yourself

Sometimes it may be more suitable for the caregiver to move in with aging parents. You may find yourself wondering if you should make this move. It all depends on how such a change will fit into your life and if you're able to incorporate it with your own commitments. You may experience feelings of resentment and anger when you move back into your parents' house if you feel that you are making a sacrifice and yet your parents react as if you're still a child living in their home.

An alternative is to move closer to your parents—into the same neighbourhood or the same apartment building. As the senior generation ages, we may see even more creative living solutions for caregivers and their families.

Assisted Living Facilities

Your parents are starting to find daily activities challenging. They require more medical care and need to have people pay closer attention to them. Perhaps your parents live alone and you are not able to visit or attend to them daily to ensure their safety. Assisted living accommodations offer nursing care and other services to help your parents in their daily routines. Often such facilities require your parents to have medical assessments

When it was time to start looking for a new home for Dad, my older sister and I researched what was around the neighbourhood. At that time it was important that he be in the same area as my sister who was taking on a large part of the care-giving role. I cannot imagine what we would have done without her level head and loving concern for Dad! She was the one who was taking him to most of his many doctors' appointments. We knew he needed to be somewhere that would be able to provide help and where people would keep an eye out when he needed any-thing. We also needed to make sure it would have wheelchair accessibility as he is using a walker now. And looking towards the future, we knew his care needs would increase, so an assisted living facility was the solution.

BARBARA

done at time of application. Some retirement homes offer assisted living on specific floors while others are strictly assisted-living accommodations.

A room in an assisted living facility can be difficult to get into quickly. Demand is high, resulting in wait times from months to years.

Long-Term Care Homes

When your parents require professional, twenty-four-hour medical care it's a critical time in your role as caregiver because your parents will rely on you to help make many of the decisions.

If your parents' medical needs have progressed slowly, you will have time to prepare and research the care options available. However, if your parent experiences a sudden medical crisis, time becomes a factor, choices are limited and the medical community drives your decisions. Be prepared for feelings of frustration, confusion and heightened emotion as you settle your parents into a long-term care facility.

It's important to remember that unless your parents are cognitively impaired, the final decision to move into a long-term care facility will be theirs.

There's no way around it: the process of moving into a long-term care home is complicated. If your parents are not in the hospital but are applying directly from home, they will require an assessment to determine if the level of care they need warrants the move. The assessment will be done by a provincial social service agency that will guide you and help you with the application and paperwork. The agency will also be an advocate for your parents. Your parents will need to be evaluated not only for the level of care required and their eligibility but also the degree of urgency. The social service agency will provide you with a list of the long-term care homes in your area for you to review.

The stairs at my aunt's house are too dangerous for my grandmother and she needs to go to an assisted care facility. She's in one temporarily and my parents and aunt still need to go every day to make sure my grandmother is getting the care she needs. My grandmother is on a three-year waiting list to get into a permanent facility. Although she is the picture of health, she is almost ninety-six and three years is an eternity at that time of life. It's taking a toll on my aunt, who has no time for a life of her own, my parents who try to help out as much as they can but it causes marital conflicts, and local grandchildren who try to help out but feel guilty because they have children and career commitments. Out-of-town family have reconciled with the fact that someone else will care for her.

CAREGIVER, BELLE RIVER, ONTARIO

The application process varies across the provinces, as do the actual names of the institutions. For example, in Saskatchewan they are referred to as special-care homes, in New Brunswick, nursing homes and in Ontario, long-term care facilities. Long-term care homes are regulated by the government, and funded by them; as a result, subsidization is not the same in each province. These homes also vary in terms of the level and type of care offered, for example, some homes do not offer dementia care. They also differ in how they are regulated and who owns them. Long-term care homes can be privately owned, owned and operated by the local government, or non-profit.

Be aware that long-term care homes also have long waiting lists of up to several months or more. Application procedures vary by province as does the management of the waiting lists.

As an example of how your parents might get into a long-term care facility, we'll look at how the procedure works in Ontario. When your parents are applying from their home, a case manager from the Community Care Access Centre (CCAC) can help them apply. Once your parents are found to be eligible, they and you can then select up to three homes, which you list on the application in order of preference. Be sure to tour the homes with your parents prior to making a selection. Your parents will need to list the type of accommodations they prefer: private room, semi-private room or basic/standard accommodation. Basic accommodation usually has two to four people and a shared bathroom. Rooms vary in price.

At this point your parents' applications are sent to the home for review and, if accepted, your parents' names will be put on the waiting list. The amount of time your parents will have to wait will vary depending on the home, the preferred accommodation and the level of care your parents require. If there are changes in your parents' health that affect their application while they are waiting, they can contact their case manager who will assess the urgency of their situation.

Your parents will be notified once a room becomes available. They will then have twenty-four-hours to decide if they will accept the room. Usually they can move in the next day. If your parents cannot move in right away, they can delay the move for up to five days but they will be charged a fee for holding the space. If your parents turn down an offer at any of the homes, they will be removed from all waiting lists and will need to wait six months before reapplying. If there is a serious change in your parents' health during the six months requiring an immediate move into long-term care, they can contact their case manager who will help them reapply. If your parents are not accepted into their preferred home, they can accept the room offered and remain on the waiting lists with the other homes.

Your parents may also apply to a long-term care facility from the hospital because their care needs do not allow them to return home. If this is the situation, your case manager will assist you and your parents, or a social worker or discharge planner from

- They are experiencing cognitive impairment.
- They are experiencing a continuing medical condition that requires close professional attention.
- Their condition doesn't allow them to live on their own.
- They have had multiple hospital admissions indicating they need additional help.
- Family or community support is not available.

the hospital will help you with the application process. Your social service agency will have more information about the application process in your province (see the Senior and Caregiver Resource Guide under Social Services Support and Assessment for contact information).

Once it's determined that your parents are going to be moving into a long-term care home, you need to research available facilities. It is important that you have visited all of the homes you list, in order to be sure you've made the right choice for your parents.

It was time to make other arrangements for my mother's safety and care. My husband, Jack, and I interviewed fifteen nursing homes and luckily got her into a well-run home with lots of caring staff. The day was May 17, 1997—to this day, the worst day of my life! That was the day we had to leave her at her new and last home. I was advised to stay away for three weeks until they settled her in; I lasted ten days. Surprisingly, she wasn't as mad at me as I had anticipated. Her big problem was that she didn't have a lock on the door; she wanted my son to come and install one. I explained they couldn't have a lock as the nurses needed twenty-four-hour access.

The next day I got a phone call from Mom asking me to see Mr. Wilson (our former lawyer who passed away thirty years ago) and get him to draw up the papers to buy the place, as it is a real money-maker! When she was younger, Mom had owned rooming houses in Toronto with forty-four tenants. When asked, I told her she owned it now and she was as pleased as punch. She would introduce me as her general manager and if they had any problems contact me. It pleased her, so it pleased me.

Her condition progressed slowly at first then advanced sooner than we hoped for. She had a fractured hip that left her in a wheelchair, but that didn't stop her getting around. To find her, I had to go on a hunt every time I went to visit. She would tell me, "Those poor old souls are lonesome and need company."

It amazed me how few people ever came to visit her. It was as if she didn't exist any more. That hurt, when I knew how kind she had been to so many people in her lifetime. One major exception was her best friend Myrtle. Myrtle had moved to Calgary and phoned and wrote Mother on a regular basis for over seventeen years, now that is loyalty!

Mom passed away quickly in her ninety-first year, with little suffering. There isn't a day goes by that we don't mention Noni in one way or another.

I consider myself the luckiest woman in the world to have had such a wonderful influence in my life, as well as being my best friend!

LYNDA, MARKHAM, ONTARIO

Part of your research should include reviewing the government inspection reports for each facility. Because long-term care homes are regulated by the government, each should have its inspection results available. The reports list safety concerns such as unsafe food preparation as well as quality-of-life standards such as available recreational activities. Requirements for inspections vary by province. They may be done annually, periodically or as a result of a complaint. Where you can find these reports varies by province. You can ask to see it while at the home, check the local library, or make a formal request to your government through the Freedom of Information Act. Ontario and Quebec post their reports online. (In our Senior and Caregiver Resource Guide, you'll find them in Ontario under the Ministry of Health and Long-Term Care and in Quebec under the Ministère de la Santé et des Services Sociaux.)

Most long-term care homes offer basic or preferred accommodation; some offer private and semi-private rooms. Most of them have a main dining area and common rooms and some also have a lounge, gift shop, beauty salon, chapel and garden. You can usually obtain a basic package that includes furnishings, meals, bed linens and laundry, personal service, housekeeping, medical supplies, medication administration and social and recreational activities. Sometimes there are optional services that you can pay for such as hairdressing,

My seventy-seven-year-old widowed mother recently had emergency bowel obstruction surgery (she'd already had three hip replacements). When we entered her home we were shocked. We found she had been living in squalor and filth for at least three years—with no running water in her kitchen. Somehow she was able to hide this from us. She is now living with us in our "granny suite" and we are trying to find her a safe place to live that she can afford. We are coping but it sure has been a challenging time.

JANE, INDIAN HEAD, SASKATCHEWAN

cable TV service and transportation. Take a checklist of questions with you when you preview each home.

PREVIEWING A LONG-TERM CARE FACILITY CHECKLIST

Financial and Administrative

- [ ] How long is the waiting list?
- [ ] What are base costs and add-ons?
- [ ] How is billing arranged? What are the extra charges if any?
- [ ] What are the visiting times?
- [ ] Can outings and overnight stays be arranged?
- [ ] Can residents bring their own food?
- [ ] Can residents bring their own furniture?
- [ ] What are practices regarding belongings, pets and mail?
- [ ] What are policies around smoking and alcoholic beverages?
- [ ] What kind of clothing should residents bring?
- [ ] Does the facility require clothing to be labelled?
- [ ] Is there an option to keep personal belongings secure?

Staff

- [ ] What is the staff-to-resident ratio?
- [ ] Are employees bonded?
- [ ] Does staff respond quickly to requests?
- [ ] Is the staff friendly? Are they willing to answer questions?
- [ ] Is there a tone of dignity and respect for the residents?
- [ ] How does the staff interact with the residents?

Health Care

- [ ] Is your family doctor able to continue to provide care?
- [ ] How does the facility control infectious outbreaks?
- [ ] Does the facility accept people with dementia?
- [ ] Are any residents restrained? And why?
- [ ] Are residents engaged or just sitting passively?
- [ ] Do residents look content and cared for?
- [ ] Are family members involved in residents' care?

Safety

- [ ] When was the last government inspection report? Request to see it.
- [ ] How often is the home inspected?
- [ ] Is the facility accredited?
- [ ] What are the emergency/fire procedures?

Services and Amenities

- [ ] What special needs can they accommodate?
- [ ] Is a social worker available if necessary?
- [ ] Is it easy for you and other family members to get to the location?
- [ ] Are there areas where family can visit privately?
- [ ] Is it able to meet religious, cultural, language and dietary needs?
- [ ] What activities are provided? Do they sound appealing?
- [ ] Is public or volunteer transportation available?
- [ ] Are there choices at mealtimes (menu, location and times)? Can you sample a meal?
- [ ] Are the meals cooked on-site or at a central kitchen, which then freezes and ships to the facility?

Facility

☐ Do you sense an atmosphere of warmth and concern?

☐ Does the facility appear clean and have good natural lighting?

☐ Is it properly ventilated to minimize unpleasant odours?

Adapted from Community Care Access Centre Ontario, "Residential Care Checklist."

Accepting that Your Parents Are Moving into Long-Term Care

Thinking about long-term care for your parents is difficult and emotional. We associate these facilities with images of illness and elderly people not having control over their lives. It's not easy to picture your parents there. It's scary to put your trust in other people to care for your parents.

Once they are settled in the long-term care home, visiting can be depressing. But it's important to move beyond these uncomfortable emotions for your parents' sake and to visit as often as possible and encourage family members to do so as well.

At this stage you are acknowledging that your parents require more than your caregiving abilities allow and likely you will feel guilt that you didn't do enough.

 We had to find a nursing home suitable for my sixty-nine-year-old father as none of his five children were in a position to care for him properly. And that is key—proper care! Too many people (including my mum) think it is their obligation to care for ailing relatives, however, family can't always provide the *best* care for the patient.

SHEILA, GRIMSBY, ONTARIO

Helping Your Parents Stay at Home for the Duration of Care

Some families wish to offer a very ill parent care within the home rather than moving them into a long-term care facility. In this case, medical care and eventually palliative care will be

I cared for my mother when she was in and out of the hospital, waking up every hour with her, tending to her every need and holding her close to me. I told her how much she was loved and what a great mother she was.

Today my mother is in a nursing home. She is now in a wheelchair, because she is too weak to walk. Sometimes she remembers my last visit and other times she does not. She calls me, when her memory serves her well, and I cannot express how my heart feels when I hear her voice, knowing that she remembered me and how her face lights up when she sees me and my daughter. I cannot help but hug her tightly and kiss her over and over again on her sweet face. Mom, I love you, and when the day comes that you no longer remember me, I know that deep in your heart we will always be mother and daughter. Ours is a love so special, a love so powerful that no illness, no cancer, no suffering can ever take it away.

CAREGIVER, TORONTO, ONTARIO

required. As your parents' health declines you will need to rely heavily on formal care through provincial health programs and the social services in your community, such as the Victorian Order of Nurses, the Canadian Red Cross and other local senior organizations, to make sure that your parents receive a high level of care. (See the Senior and Caregiver Resource Guide for more information.)

A Place to Call Home

It's not easy to watch your parents need more care and have to move out of their home. You are dealing with your own emotions while helping your parents adjust to a new environment and lifestyle. Strive to help them feel comfortable and happy no matter where they are living.

During this time the importance of communication—with your parents, family members and the various social agencies and medical personnel—cannot be underestimated. It's essential to ensure you have all the right information to help make informed decisions, and that all decisions are discussed with your parents and other involved family members. Remember that your goal is to care for your parents in a way that maintains their dignity and independence while providing comfort and safety.

My mother made the most unusual decision while she was recovering in the hospital last summer. She told me that she was tired of cooking and wanted to move directly into a long-term care facility in her hometown. "Great," I said. "We'll arrange for an interview with the hospital administrator who facilitates these applications and go from there." She had to choose three locations, and after that was done (along with lots of paperwork) she then waited and waited in the long-term care wing of the small-town hospital. After six months and much frustration with a room-mate who would wake her in the middle of the night, she got her call. It happened two days after Christmas and was the best gift. She was notified that she would be moving into her first choice and she had a private room. She was thrilled.

My mother was born in the 1920s to a large farm family. She met a young soldier during the war and corresponded with him while he crossed the country. They married in 1945. They lived and worked a farm together for sixty years until he died. She stayed in the farm-house another year; she liked her own company but I knew she felt housebound during that first winter alone. She would spend a few weeks with me in Toronto. We had such fun. At the age of eighty-two she had her first manicure. She went to the top of the CN

Tower. She had her hair cut and styled. She shopped for her own clothes. She said yes to everything!

Now she is having a great time in her new digs. After three years of being my father's full-time nurse, she is now able to do some relaxing. Although, her usual response to "How are things?" is "I'm busy, busy, busy." At the nursing home there is always something to do or someone coming in to entertain the group. During this past long snowy winter she hasn't been housebound, she has been out-bound. Her social life has been transformed.

Truly I have felt relieved of the guilt of trying to visit her frequently. On a good day, it's a three-hour round trip, and with my husband working on the east coast I am basically a single parent with a demanding job and a wonderful son who is busy.

She and my father were an inspiration. They were always out and about visiting people, dropping in without an invitation (not like we city folk, where you have to make an appointment a week in advance to visit a friend). The visiting was to ensure that their friends were healthy and to keep in touch, oh, and to have a cup of tea and a slice of pie perhaps. I am so glad that my mother is in a place where she can walk safely around the hallways dropping in on others for a quick visit, and in the summer she'll have the gardens to enjoy.

JANET JOY, TORONTO, ONTARIO

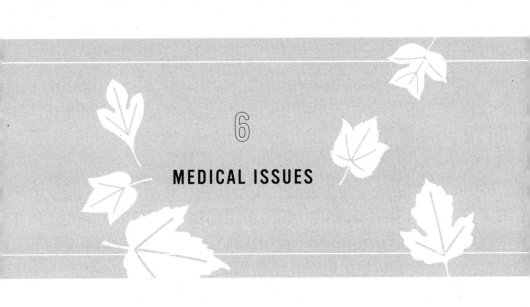

6

MEDICAL ISSUES

Being involved with your parents' health is going to be one of the largest and most important parts of your caregiving responsibilities and you may be surprised and even daunted by the quantity of information to sift through and access. This chapter will give you information about

- helping your parents stay healthy
- the importance of keeping watch and having open dialogue
- how to manage information
- tips for dealing with your parents' medications
- appointments with your parents' doctors
- medical conditions associated with aging
- geriatric assessments
- hospital visits and palliative care.

The natural aging process will bring about changes in your parents' physical well-being, and in their early senior years, your role as caregiver will be to pay attention to these changes and address any that might lead to problems. As your parents age and especially as they enter their later senior years, you will have to be more proactive, assisting them with decision-making and necessary adjustments, and communicating with their doctors.

You may find it difficult to develop an open dialogue with your parents about their health, something they may consider a very private matter. At the same time you will be challenged emotionally; it's not easy to watch your parents decline physically. If and when your parents develop more serious or complicated health issues, many of your decisions will be guided by doctors and other health professionals. You will need to increase your knowledge base while at the same time learn to rely on others' expertise. It's important that you find professionals you and your parents can trust. For as long as you can, you will help your parents to make the best choices possible, and eventually, if they cannot, you will have to make them yourself.

Keeping Your Parents Healthy

Good physical and mental health affects whether your parents want to and are able to participate in family outings and in community activities. At the same time, socializing itself can promote health, so the benefits work both ways. Encourage your parents to stay active, to exercise their minds and bodies. To keep their minds active, suggest that they do crossword puzzles or read, or start recording the family history or their memoirs. Or suggest that they take up a new activity. At the very least, encourage walking, which has been shown to have health benefits. Consider accompanying your parents on a weekly walk, both to encourage them in the exercise and as an opportunity to spend time with them.

It's important to your parents' health that they remain socially active. Help them to stay in touch with family and friends, people they care about. They can also get involved in senior community centres and day programs (some are culturally oriented, which may make your parents more comfortable).

Socializing helps prevent the loneliness and depression that can threaten people as they age.

When and How to Get Involved

Being aware of your parents' health is an essential part of caregiving. Learn what is normal for them now, how they respond to everyday aches and pains, and how they identify when something more serious is going on with them physically. Develop an open dialogue with your parents so that they are comfortable talking to you about any health issues they may have. Fear of poor health is something many of us, not just the aged, experience. Your parents may not be willing to tell you if they feel sick; talking to you means having to admit

As seniors age, routine increasingly becomes important. Be aware that your parents can easily become confused when their routine changes.

something is the matter and deal with it. Worse yet, they may not even realize when something is wrong, so sometimes you may have to play detective. Or your parents may not be telling you everything because they don't want to inconvenience or burden you.

When calling or visiting, ask questions about how they are feeling. Really listen to their answers. Pay attention to physical changes. Problems in their ability to carry out everyday activities can be symptoms of more serious issues.

One way to keep up to date on your parents' health is to offer to accompany them to their doctors' appointments. If they do not want you to go into the office with them, driving them to the appointment can be the first step, and a good opportunity to casually learn more about their health. During the drive there, ask how they are feeling, and on the drive back, how the doctor visit went. Gradually become familiar with the doctor and nurses in the office, so that they know you are available if and when the time comes that you need to become more involved in your parents' care.

Encourage your parents to have regular medical checkups, as well as hearing and eyesight examinations. Actively research any illnesses they already have, to gain a better understanding of these and in order to recognize signs of improvement or decline. If your parents are currently healthy, educate yourself about the most common ailments of seniors to help with early detection. (See page 143 for a list of common ailments, and our Senior and Caregiver Resource Guide for contact information for a number of specialized health organizations.)

How You Manage Information

Dealing with your parents' medical care can be stressful and frustrating, especially in a crisis. You need information in order to make informed decisions, but sometimes you will feel that you have too much information, and other times not enough. One day things will move too quickly and you don't have enough time to think through a decision; another day it may seem that developments are taking too long, that you're not getting the information you need as quickly as you should. Being prepared will help to reduce the anxiety and fear that can overwhelm you when dealing with the medical system.

Depending on your personality, you may find it difficult to ask questions of doctors, but it's important to speak up if something is unclear to you or if you feel you need more information. Recognize that not all doctors are the same; some are better than others at communicating. Especially in the hospital, doctors may seem too busy to answer your questions. But keep asking: the more informed you feel, the more confident you will be when making decisions.

Some of the information you need will change as your parents' health problems advance. Prioritize by deciding what information is relevant and what you can file away for future use, or disregard completely. People, your parents included, differ in how much they want to know. You may find that your parents want as much information as possible right away, or alternatively, that they are more comfortable knowing information only when they require it to make a decision.

Recognizing how much information your parents want and how they respond to it will help you find the best way to communicate with them about medical issues, lessen frustration on both sides, and be more effective as caregiver. And recognizing how you yourself process information will affect how you communicate with the doctors, what kind of research you do and how you discuss medical developments with your parents.

Medications

Your parents may take a number of medications at any given point for different conditions. You can help make it easier for them to take medications appropriately and safely by putting a couple of simple systems in place.

ORGANIZE MEDICATIONS

In the early stages of caregiving you may feel that your parents are capable of managing their medicine, but you should always be aware of what they are taking and watch for indicators that they are having problems. If you find that they require help, review with your parents all the medications they have been prescribed. Together you should review them so that you know when the medications should be taken and if there are any special instructions. Oftentimes our parents are taking several pills a day. No wonder they get confused!

Pillboxes can help you organize the pills by day of the week and time. There are a variety of these available at your local drugstore. Another option is to have the pharmacy divide your parents' prescriptions into prepared packets by dosage, days and times of day. Most pharmacies offer this service; check with your parents' pharmacy to see what is available.

Remembering when to take medications can be challenging for seniors. Pillboxes not only help your parents to organize their medications but also are a helpful reminder tool, preventing under- or overmedication. By glancing at the boxes, they can easily see whether they have taken their pills for a certain day or time.

USE REMINDER AIDS FOR MEDICATION

Setting up simple reminder aids can help your parents, regardless of their age, to feel that they are still able to do things for themselves, allowing them to maintain their sense of personal dignity and to feel satisfaction in their achievements. Although for you dealing with everyday decisions and errands may seem mundane, for your parents these can be life affirming.

> Every Saturday my dad sorts his pills for the week into his pill containers. It's a slow process and takes him time to make sure it's done right. Afterwards, my sister checks to make sure everything is where it should be. One of us could do it quicker, but it's important that he still does it in his own time for as long as he's able to.
>
> BARBARA

Beyond pillboxes, another good way for your parents to remember to take their medication is to connect it with a regular daily activity. For example, if they have to take a certain pill in the morning, they might remember to do so if it's associated with brushing their teeth.

If you notice that your parents are forgetting to take medication, look into purchasing an alarm timer (Barbara's dad uses one). These devices beep to alert the user that it's time to take medication.

Another reminder method is to post a medication chart somewhere within sight, such as on the fridge door. These charts list the medication by time and day, and as your parents take each dosage they cross it off. Such charts are a good way for you as caregiver to monitor medications as well as any changes in your parents' short-term memory. It's a good idea to write a description beside the medication name. If it's a pill, what colour is it? What size is it? This helps your to remember which pill they are supposed to take.

TALK TO YOUR PARENTS' PHARMACIST

Put aside time to talk to your parents' pharmacist about all the medications that they are taking. A pharmacist can review their medications and let you know which ones can be taken together (and which ones cannot). Taking medication fewer times each day will reduce the chances of your parents forgetting to take them. Ask the pharmacist what you should do if they do forget to take some, or if they take too much. Don't forget to mention any over-the-counter or herbal remedies your parents may be taking to make sure these are not interfering with anything prescribed. The pharmacist can also let you know how certain medications will interact with one another, and about any possible side effects. In Ontario, your provincial health plan will cover a thirty-minute appointment with your pharmacist to review medications. Such appointments must be booked ahead.

Also ask your pharmacist how you can dispose of medications that your parents are no longer taking or that have expired. Most pharmacies will take care of these if you drop them off. Do not keep these medications around the house. The fewer pill bottles there are around your parents' home, the less confusing

TIPS FOR ORGANIZING MEDICATIONS

- Request additional prescription labels be printed in large type and provided to your parents.
- Encourage your parents to take their medications where there is lots of light, so that they can see the pills clearly.
- Suggest that they keep glasses or a magnifying glass where they typically take their medications.
- Check whether their medications are available in other forms that they might find easier to take: capsules, tablets or fluid. If your parents find it difficult to open childproof lids, ask the pharmacy to use regular lids. **Caution:** if there are children around, these must be kept in a safe place.
- Review with your parents every three months how their medications are to be taken: with water or food, swallowed or chewed, at night or in the morning.
- Put a system in place to alert you and your parents when prescription refills or renewals are needed. A doctor visit may be required for renewals; planning ahead will allow you to fit the visit into your schedule. Some drugstores now have automatic renewal reminder systems by e-mail or by phone.

it will be for them, and the less likely it is that they'll accidentally take the wrong medication.

Your Relationship with the Family Doctor

Develop a relationship with your parents' doctor. Your parents may want you to sit in on the appointments, which is ideal, or you may have to ask them if they are comfortable with your presence.

Attending an appointment can be helpful if your parents are finding it hard to remember what to ask the doctor during the session, or what the doctor says in order to convey it to you later. Often seniors have trouble hearing what is said, or become confused. When accompanying your parents, take a notebook of questions to ask the doctors and note recommendations they make.

You and your parents may need to schedule a special appointment with the doctor if you want a complete review of their current situation. When you sit in with your parents on this visit, take the opportunity to review your parents' medications. Ask why each one has been prescribed. Also check with the doctor about your parents' medical conditions, asking what symptoms to expect and how you can tell if their condition is worsening.

Ask your parents to talk to their doctors and identify you as their caregiver. They should let doctors know that you are interested in receiving any information they feel is pertinent. If your parents are hospitalized and unable to tell the doctors to include you in any decision-making, whoever has power of attorney for personal care will work with the doctors. (See page 168 for a definition of power of attorney.)

If your parents are refusing to include you in their doctor's visits, due to doctor-patient confidentiality the doctor may not talk directly to you. You should continue to try to communicate with your parents about their health. If you are concerned about a specific behaviour or symptom you could call your parents' doctor and let him or her know so they are aware and can observe on your parents' next visit. If you feel the situation is critical and your parents are in danger, you may need to have the person who has been assigned the power of attorney for personal care step in.

Communication with the family doctor is crucial. Remember to pay attention and listen carefully to what he or she says. To be of help to your parents, you need to keep an open mind

CREATE A PERSONAL MEDICAL
NOTEBOOK FOR YOUR PARENTS

A personal medical notebook contains your parents' personal information, medical history and medications. It is important because it

- contains your parents' dates of birth, health insurance numbers, address, phone number and details of third-party medical coverage
- records medications, drug interactions and allergies
- records medical procedures and important dates
- is useful if someone other than the caregiver needs to take your parents to an appointment
- provides a record of treatments and conversations if your parents see multiple doctors
- can be taken along to record what is discussed in a doctor visit, or to provide information to the doctor
- allows everyone in the family to stay up to date.

about the information the doctor is giving you, even if it is not what you want to hear, or expect to hear. For the benefit of your parents, you must be willing to deal with difficult news, and to help them deal with this news too. If this is emotional for you, imagine how it feels to them. Your ability to move past your own fears in order to ask questions, and really listen to the answers, is key to making the right choices for your parents' health.

HAVE INFORMATION AVAILABLE

When visiting with a doctor or in case of an emergency you should have relevant information at hand in order to save time and prevent confusion (not to mention more stress). Remember to bring your parents' personal medical notebook (see previous page) in case you have to help them fill out forms.

Your parents should also keep a copy of their personal details and a list of current medications in a wallet or a purse in case of an emergency. Keep a full list of medications somewhere accessible, such as on your parents' fridge, so that in an emergency attendants have the details at hand. Check with your parents' pharmacy as many of them now print out descriptions of a patient's medications in various sizes.

I noticed that going for a doctor appointment has changed. I used to drive to the plaza, drop him near the door, and come back and pick him up. Then I started going in with him in case he needed help filling out the papers. I would wait in the reception area for him. Now I arrive at his residence about forty-five minutes early. He is usually ready to go but I casually check out his clothes, making sure everything is in order.

I have a mental checklist that includes wallet, OHIP card, list of pills, any necessary paperwork, any pills that he needs to take during the time we will be away, and water. Once we're ready to leave, it's a long and slow walk down the hall.

Inevitably when we're at the elevator Dad will mention he needs his cap. "Wait here, I'll go back to your room and get it." Now we're ready to leave. Dad waits at the door, while I get the car. I watch him carefully getting into the car and then I put the walker into the trunk. I'm already thinking, will we get there on time? We usually do arrive on time, then I do the checking in and we both go into the office together. I'm always hoping they don't send us for lab tests because these appointments seem to get longer and longer.

JOAN, TORONTO, ONTARIO

QUESTIONS TO ASK THE DOCTOR ABOUT MEDICATIONS

- What is the name of the medication?
- Why do your parents need to take it?
- How should they take it?
- What are the side effects?
- What do your parents do when they run out?
- Where should they keep it?
- If they forget to take it at the usual time, can they take it later in the day or should they skip it?
- What do they do with medications that they no longer need?

Also on the fridge your parents should keep a list of local walk-in clinics as a backup in case their doctor is not available, and a list of nearby labs for blood tests or X-rays, along with hours these are open. Although this may seem like a lot of information to post, in an emergency these lists will save time and effort for your parents, you as caregiver, or anyone else helping them.

Attending Specialist Doctor Appointments

In addition to visiting the family doctor with your parents, at some stage you will likely need to go to specialist appointments. Often the waits for these appointments are very long, and they almost always involve your parents' getting tests or blood work done. Make sure your parents do what is necessary to prepare. Usually the receptionist will give you instructions prior to the test: take medications or not, fast or not. If you're going to see a doctor in a hospital for the first time and don't have the required hospital card, leave home early so you have time to register.

Can someone survive congestive heart failure in their eighties? Apparently so. ICU visit, signing wills at the bedside, pastoral visits, family on alert, but slowly and surely recovery happens. With Dad in hospital and Mom unable to be alone, I take leave from work to stay with her. We drive to the hospital daily to sit by the bedside so they can hold hands. "When can he come home?" the question is repeated endlessly.

The day Dad is discharged from the hospital, we cheerfully head home. Dad is tired. He sleeps most of the day. He gets up to eat; he falls asleep in the chair during dinner. He lives in the bed. For the first week, we must arrive at the outpatient clinic at 7 a.m. for blood tests so medication can be adjusted. Getting up and moving at that hour with an eighty-year-old—coordinating transportation, getting dressed, eating some food—is mayhem. (Who makes these rules?) We get through the testing period, and settle into a routine of waking him to take medication twice a day.

Back in Ottawa, I call regularly to see how they are. Everything is fine, they report, with rather forced cheerfulness. My brother reports Dad's blood clotting is not at a good level. Too high a clotting level can lead to a heart attack or stroke, too low and the heart works inefficiently. Seems the medications are not being taken. My dad was always the one to watch that they both took their meds. Now many medications remain at the end of the week. The pre-measured blister packs have many unopened doors. If my dad is not compliant with his medications the doctor indicates we cannot continue to treat the condition. A caregiver is hired to go in every day for a few hours. One of her responsibilities is to ensure they take their morning medications. Negotiations with the doctor and pharmacist finally lead to all essential medications being prepared in the morning dose.

"Did you take your medications," each of us asks as we visit or phone, especially on weekends when the caregiver does not go in.

"Yes, don't worry," is the reply. Sometimes, "That's all you think about," or "You remind me of my mother."

Meanwhile spot checks reveal that when no one watches medications are not taken. Weekends pass, blood work is out of line. Sigh. My brother makes a scheduled visit each weekend morning. We give up on evening meds, which remain sporadically taken at best. Sharing our story with friends reveals we are not alone. There is comfort in that.

MARIANNE, OTTAWA, ONTARIO

Also, remember your parents' medical history notebook as they may be asked about medications as well as past medical procedures and surgeries and their approximate dates. Be aware that often specialists don't consult with each other, and one might ask you for information about visits to other specialists.

Specialist appointments may feel rushed, so prepare your questions in advance, especially as there may not be a follow-up appointment. It's natural that your feelings of stress, and those of your parents, will heighten as medical issues become more complicated. Try not to let yourself get flustered or intimidated.

Ask the doctor questions about what to expect with the illness and what treatment options are viable. Knowing the positives and negatives of certain treatments will help you and your parents to weigh their options. Discuss whether diet and exercise affects the illness (they often do). Take notes, and write down the name of the illness, checking the spelling so that you can do further research at home. Ask for clarification if there's any medical jargon that you don't understand. Ask whether it's necessary to book follow-up appointments. Make the appointment before you leave or take a card with you to remember to phone when you get home. Ask whether there's anything more you can do to help your parents.

Maintaining Your Parents' Dignity at Appointments

During a doctor visit your parents may need assistance undressing or getting up on the exam table. Getting them settled comfortably before the doctor arrives will help them maintain their personal dignity. If your parents are not feeling flustered and disorganized, they will feel more confident and have a sense of control when speaking with the doctor. Give your parents the chance to express how they are feeling to you and the doctor in the appointments.

Communicating with Your Parents After the Appointment

When you talk with your parents about medical issues, don't use the medical jargon that the doctor may have used. Use plain language, without being condescending, then ask them to repeat what you told them to make sure they understand, especially if it's regarding medication or treatments. Organize the information into clear, concise points. If they don't seem to understand, rephrase what you said. Be supportive and remember to listen to your parents' opinions and feelings. When you arrive home from doctor's appointments take time to review instructions, organize medications and write down any important information so they have it for reference. Offer your parents an action plan of things they can do to deal with the condition as effectively as possible. This will help them to feel more in control.

Medical Conditions Associated with Aging

As your parents age they may experience any number of common illnesses. Recognizing early symptoms of these diseases can help you to know when to step in as caregiver and offer assistance.

To name a few, your parents may face arthritis, foot problems, hearing loss, heart disease, osteoporosis, stroke, diabetes, deteriorating vision, dementia, incontinence, anxiety, depression, loneliness, cancer, memory loss and sleeping problems. And they may experience several of these health issues in the early stages of aging. As caregiver you should watch for symptoms of these conditions, and also any indication that they are becoming more serious.

SYMPTOMS ASSOCIATED WITH COMMON ILLNESSES

- Heart disease: weakness, fatigue, shortness of breath
- Diabetes: changes in appetite, weight loss or gain, sores that don't heal well, changes in eyesight, constant drinking and urination
- Osteoporosis: loss of height or hunching, frequent bone breaks
- Cancer: sudden weight loss or pain
- Stroke: difficulty with speech, loss of feeling in one side, confusion
- Depression: lack of motivation to tackle daily activities, reduced socializing, feelings of loneliness

Just because your parents exhibit symptoms doesn't mean that they have the condition, but if you notice any of these developments, have them visit their family doctor.

MEMORY LOSS

As your parents age they may become increasingly forgetful. This could be a simple sign of growing older or it could be a symptom of dementia, such as Alzheimer's disease (see page 147 for symptoms). If you notice that they are forgetting the odd appointment, encourage them to keep a calendar high-lighting special events, doctor appointments and family birth-days. Call them routinely to remind them about certain daily or weekly tasks they should perform, such as taking the garbage out. Try not to get frustrated when they tell you the same story over and over; just gently remind them you already know the story, or else be patient, recognizing that they are sharing their life stories with you.

HEARING LOSS

If you find yourself often repeating things to your parents, it's probably time to have their hearing tested. Hearing loss can be remedied quite easily with a hearing aid. Some seniors are resistant to this idea, however, and may have to have the bene-fits of better hearing through an aid pointed out to them by a professional.

When you are out with your parents be aware that others may perceive them as being rude and ignoring them when in reality they are having hearing problems. Hearing loss can also impact their safety when they are out walking, or driving a car.

STRESS AND ANXIETY

Experiencing stress and anxiety during the aging process are not unusual; after all, your parents are going through many changes, both physical and emotional. One way to help your parents over-come these feeling is to encourage them to maintain a healthy level of physical and social activity. Suggest that they go for a walk around the block to get some fresh air. Maybe they can take an exercise class for seniors. Get them involved in an activity they enjoy doing, or encourage them to take time to relax and read a book or listen to music. They can talk to a friend or family mem-ber, or you as caregiver, about how they are feeling. You may be able to help simply by listening, but if that doesn't work, suggest that they talk to a doctor, see a counsellor or join a support group.

SLEEP PROBLEMS

As people age they often find it difficult to sleep or require less sleep. Your parents may think this is their problem alone, but in fact it is common among seniors. Linda's mom was advised by her doctor not to nap in the afternoon as it would affect her ability to sleep at night. As a result, she would run her errands during the afternoon. If your parents complain of not being able to sleep well, suggest one of the following strategies:

- Get up and do something else for a while and then go back to bed.
- Drink warm milk or hot water with lemon before bed.
- Get fresh air and exercise during the day.
- Take a warm bath, read a little or listen to music before bed.
- Go to bed and get up at the same time every day to maintain a routine.
- Don't drink coffee, tea, soda or alcohol in the evening.
- Don't take naps during the day.

Some medications affect sleep patterns, so sleep problems may be due to medication type or dosage; have your parents speak to their doctor about this side effect. If they complain about other physical symptoms such as pain, anxiety or depression, this is a more serious health issue that may require medical attention.

LONELINESS AND DEPRESSION

Your parents may start to feel lonely as they age. They may experience the loss of other elderly family members, friends, or their spouse, which can lead to depression. Try to visit as often as possible and encourage other family members and friends to do so too. Have your parents take the initiative and call to talk to a friend or family member every day. Keeping busy helps. Perhaps your parents can volunteer at a local school, church or community centre. Or they can join a senior club and get involved in an activity they enjoy doing, or learn something new.

While experiencing periods of sadness and loneliness is natural, if you find your parents are experiencing the symptoms below they may be suffering from clinical depression and they should see their doctor.

SYMPTOMS OF CLINICAL DEPRESSION

The primary symptom of depression is a sad and hopeless mood that occurs most days and lasts for more than two weeks. This mood affects the ability to carry out daily functions and to socialize. Other symptoms include:

- changes in appetite and weight
- problems sleeping
- lost interest in hobbies and daily activities
- withdrawal from family and friends
- feelings of uselessness, excessive guilt and a pessimistic outlook
- agitation and distress
- lethargy
- irritability and tiredness
- trouble concentrating or making decisions
- crying for no reason or being unable to cry
- thoughts of suicide
- delusional thinking.

DEMENTIA

One of the most heartbreaking and difficult diseases to cope with as children and caregivers to our parents is dementia. It's hard to accept that your parents as you once knew them are slipping away from you. If they exhibit symptoms of memory loss, aggression and confusion, talk to their doctor. You will need to arrange a geriatric assessment to determine what stage your parents are at. Dementia is not only hard on your parents but extremely hard for family members and friends.

ALZHEIMER'S DISEASE[13]

Here is a list of symptoms that may indicate Alzheimer's disease:

- memory loss that affects day-to-day function
- difficulty performing familiar tasks
- problems with language
- disorientation in time or place
- poor or decreased judgment
- problems with abstract thinking
- misplacing of items
- changes in mood and behaviour
- changes in personality
- loss of initiative.

The Safely Home program is a national, fee-based service that allows you to register your parents in case they wander and forget their way home. It is run by the Alzheimer Society of Canada in conjunction with the RCMP. Those who register are issued a bracelet with a registration number that links them to a national database that can be accessed by the RCMP. Visit this website for more information: www.safelyhome.ca.

Geriatric Assessments

A geriatric assessment is a series of tests that help evaluate a senior's mental and physical condition. The assessment allows your parents' doctors to determine how to improve their quality of life and allow them to live as independently as possible.

Your parents' family doctor will give your parents a referral to get the assessment if he or she feels it's necessary. You can also request a referral if your parents show signs of memory loss, confusion or other possible symptoms of dementia, or if there is a sudden decline in their ability to function, or they have extreme behavioural changes and multiple medical issues. The assessment can determine if their symptoms are those of dementia or the result of an interaction between medications.

Geriatric assessments are usually performed by a gerontologist, who may involve other doctors such as a neurologist and a psychologist. The appointment is usually arranged such that your parents visit one doctor after another on the same day, and because of this the test is generally carried out at a hospital.

If your parents are to go through this testing, talk to them in advance so that they are aware of what is involved. The test includes a physical and mental health exam, and will help determine your parents' ability to perform basic activities of daily living. It will also evaluate their living arrangements, social network and access to support services, and help to identify current problems and potential future ones.

Using the results of the assessment, the doctors will help you as the caregiver to develop a care plan, including making recommendations for support services. The assessment can help to make the interaction more efficient among your parents, involved family members and community resources. It also sets in motion a system of ongoing monitoring that will evaluate changes in your parents in the future.

It started about five years ago. My father had his first stroke, [and] we went through the first few weeks of him having massive confusion and difficulty swallowing. He went to rehab and was quite manageable for the next two years. When he had his second stroke, his personality and his demands on my mother took a toll on her. She is now a prisoner in her own home, suffering from depression and anxiety. We have recently started the process of trying to place him in a home but we are all feeling guilty about it.

My mom is afraid to be alone if he goes to a nursing home. She has taken on the role of wife, caregiver, mother and god-sent angel. I am afraid for her own health and well-being. When is it time to say "let the responsibility go"? Or is that what is keeping her going?

He still suffers from more mini-strokes. His conversations are very hard to understand. His patience is short and his thoughts are irrational. Who will be the one he hates for placing him in a home?

DOREEN, FALHER, ALBERTA

As well as being part of your parents' general medical care, an assessment is also used in a medical crisis to determine if your parents are capable of returning to their home and living independently. In the future it can also be used by the family to decide whether they need to invoke the power of attorney for personal care.

Emergency Hospital Visits and Admittance

It's not easy to manoeuvre through the Canadian medical system. In fact, taking your parents to the hospital can be one of your most stressful experiences as a caregiver. And remember that it's stressful for your parents as well; it's not part of their routine, and they may get confused and find it hard to answer questions from medical staff. Try to make your parents as comfortable as possible. Remain calm and focused, offer them support and reassurance, and help them to understand what the doctors are saying.

In the hospital environment you will have to become an advocate for your parents. Ask whatever questions you feel necessary in order to understand what is happening and what is going to happen. Work *with* the doctor. You are all on the same side in trying to determine the best care for your parents. Expect a lot of waiting. You'll need to be patient and persistent at the same time.

If your parents are admitted to hospital, you should get to know the hospital staff and their schedules. Be aware of hospital procedures and policies. Check visiting hours so that you can advise family and friends. Be kind and friendly to the nurses and staff to show them that you want to be cooperative and appreciate their attention. Ask when the doctors do their rounds so that you will know when to be present to talk to them. Have questions prepared to ask them. Take notes. Know what treatment options are available to your parents, and the pros and cons of each. If your parents are coherent, try to decide together on the best course of action. Even if your parents are having a hard time communicating, continue to involve them as much as possible in discussions. Encourage other family members to come and help, to give you a chance to refresh.

Familiarize yourself with discharge procedures for the hospital. Sometimes if the hospital is busy, you will need to advocate for your parents to ensure the proper discharge procedures are followed. Your parents' physical abilities, living conditions and access to help should be evaluated before they are discharged, in case further in-home services need to be arranged.

I guess I would call my journey with my mom and dad (who are both still alive) bittersweet. We've come close to the end of the line a few times and I've believed that my mom would not make it through the night. How would I go on? How could I possibly cope? Will I, with extreme guilt, feel that a huge burden has been lifted off my shoulders? Will I feel that I am finally free to live my own life after years of living theirs? It's been so long since I've had control over my own life; would I even know what to do with myself? Both my parents are seventy-nine years old. They are both very sick in their own ways and fighting separate issues. They also both have very different personalities, which sometimes make them both impossible, and sometimes I just laugh in spite of it all.

You eventually give up your life, your comfort, your privacy, your sanity, your everything, when you take on the challenge of caring for your parents. And I'm not talking about sticking them in some nursing home and maybe visiting at holidays. I'm talking about doing everything in your power to keep them healthy and happy. I'm talking about monthly hospital visits, waiting in the emergency for ten hours at a time questioning our failing health care system. I'm talking about being their voice, their ears, their support.

Nothing tears my heart more than seeing that poor, little, lost soul, who is confused and scared and all alone in a world they can no longer understand. The ones that have no one to take care of them. That's gut-wrenching. I always tell my parents that they are so lucky to not be that person.

LORI, KITCHENER, ONTARIO

If your parents are extremely ill they will have to be assessed to determine whether they can return home safely. Or your parents may be too sick to go home and need to go to a rehabilitation centre or need to wait for a nursing home space to become available, or they may require palliative care.

Agencies and Support Organizations

If your parents are diagnosed with a medical condition, there are illness-specific organizations that can provide you with information and guide you in dealing with the medical community. These organizations can also direct you to support groups and seminars, and offer other tools to help you and your parents. (See the National section of the Senior and Caregiver Resource Guide for a listing of these organizations.)

As well, don't forget to check with your own employer to see if they offer any counselling and referral services through your benefit provider.

Palliative Care

There may come a time when your focus as a caregiver will change from finding a cure for what ails your parents to providing comfort as they draw closer to the end of their lives. This is the purpose of palliative care. At this time, your priority will be to maintain their comfort and dignity as you and they face this new reality.

Palliative care involves pain management and pain alleviation. Efforts are made to reduce symptoms such as nausea, loss of appetite and confusion. Another important aspect of palliative care is caregiver support including respite care. Palliative care also helps the family work through this difficult time of losing a loved one, through psychological, emotional and spiritual support.

Many professionals are involved in palliative care: doctors, in-home care nurses, social workers, counsellors, pharmacists, therapists and volunteer workers.

The Canadian Hospice Palliative Care Association is a good source for listings of services by provinces (see our Senior and Caregiver Resource Guide for contact details).

Help is also offered through community services and support organizations connected to specific diseases. Such help can be offered in one of several different settings depending on which you feel is the most appropriate for your parents: at home, in long-term care facilities, in hospitals with specialized units, and in hospices.

I never thought life would reverse itself. My loving mom took care of me half my life. Since my dad passed away when I was one, she has been my best friend. A few years back she was diagnosed with cancer and is now palliative, struggling day by day not wanting to let go ... of me.

I find myself caring for her as a mom would care for her child. Life has a strange way of turning around. As hard as it is every day watching her wither away, I wonder if I want her to fight or let go so peace can abide her, and pain can leave her. Is it selfish, I wonder at times, to want her to hang on?

I silence my pain and smile every day to show the world I'm okay, and I am strong, but inside I'm burning with pain, despair and heartache. What will I do when she is gone? I ask myself. I am alone and trying to cope with the fact that any day now I will lose the most important person in my entire life.

CAREGIVER, BRAMPTON, ONTARIO

> If anyone reading this is an employer of someone caring for aging parents, I hope they give some thought to the ups and downs that person may be going through. Long nights at hospitals, demanding days on their days off caring for two households, the emotional impact of the care and watching a loved one get sicker and sicker. I hope they can be a little more caring than my employer! As for the families, please try to work together. We did it. We are closer now than ever, and the time has finally come that we can live for ourselves.
>
> JANET, NANAIMO,
> BRITISH COLUMBIA

Some people feel more comfortable providing care to and making decisions for their aging parents at home than in an outside setting. When providing palliative care at home you can set up a support system to help you care for your parents, including arranging for twenty-four-hour response teams. Twenty-four-hour response teams help with urgent needs, usually on a short-term basis, that otherwise may require admission to a hospital. These teams can include a palliative care nurse and a counsellor. However, your parents may require more intense medical attention that requires them to remain in a hospital setting.

Financial assistance for palliative care varies across the country, and can depend on whether you are looking after your parents in a hospital setting or at home. If your parents are at home, you can explore whether your province offers assistance through a home-care program. Often, only a limited amount of financial support is available for services and equipment. Your parents may also have private insurance. If they are in a long-term facility, generally the cost of palliative care is covered by their fees. To determine the best place for your parents to receive palliative care, you need to take into account your financial situation.

Deciding where your parents should live when they're receiving palliative care is a tough decision that requires you to think about how much care they need and whether you can realistically provide this at home. The best setting for your parents and your family as you enter this life-altering time is a very personal choice.

Compassionate Care Leave

Caregiving affects our personal and professional lives, and as a result government and businesses are recognizing the need to assist families with aging parents. The employment standards legislation in Canada provides for a compassionate care leave. This varies slightly by province and directly relates to the impending passing of your parents. You must apply for it, so

> I could come home and talk to her about anything: my worries, stress, work, children and husband, and she would always have an answer that would make me laugh and see the positive side to every problem. My mother's last three months in the hospital were very hard and painful. Every day I would go see her at tea time. We would have a cup of tea and talk about the day when she would get through it all and come home. I would end the evening putting cream on her legs, arms and face, and she would say, "God blessed me with a daughter."
>
> Even through all her pain, she always made sure her hospital companions were looked after too. They called her the angel. Near the end it was heartbreaking as the medication she was on and the morphine they had to give her made her confused. She knew I was there but she didn't know which day or time we were in. She explained that there was a train and everyone she cared about was on it and going for a ride with her. When my mom passed away she wanted everyone around her, but she made sure I was holding her hand.
>
> MARIA, MISSISSAUGA, ONTARIO

consult with your human resource manager, who should be able to guide you through the process. Some companies also have an Employment Insurance compassionate care benefit. Check with your employer to see what options may be available to you.

Being well informed is vital to managing your parents' healthcare. Preparation is also critical when looking at our next topic of discussion: the caregiver's role with finances and legal matters.

7

FINANCIAL AND LEGAL ISSUES

As caregiver for your aging parents you will eventually become involved in helping them pay bills, as well as assisting with daily activities that involve money, such as grocery shopping, and arranging for in-home services. The time may come when you need to take charge of your parents' finances completely. In this chapter we will

- help streamline your parents' banking with automated banking options
- give you tips to help protect your parents from theft and financial abuse
- define and discuss the importance of power of attorney documents
- highlight the importance of having a will
- look at what you will need to know when your parents die.

Managing Finances

As your parents age there are some steps you can take to streamline and protect their finances in order to make things easier for you and them.

BANKING SERVICES

When your parents reach their senior years, one of the first things they should do is inquire whether their banking institution offers senior accounts. As the population ages, some banks are doing away with accounts geared toward seniors, but others continue to have them and even enhance them. Encourage your parents to compare banks to see if others offer services that will help them to lower their expenses.

The Financial Consumer Agency of Canada was established to protect and educate consumers about money. They offer tips on banking, mortgages, credit cards and more. On their website, www.fcac.gc.ca, there is a section about "The Cost of Banking," in which they provide an overview of the various banks and their services, including which ones offer senior accounts and what these entail. It's a great place to start if your parents want to compare services. The website of your parents' current bank will also have information about its senior services.

Do your parents have a complaint or question about their bank? All banks are required to have a system in place to handle customer inquiries. Most banks have their own ombudsman to

BANKING FOR SENIORS

Many seniors' accounts offer

- zero monthly fees
- no minimum account balance required to receive zero monthly fees
- no fees, or lower fees on regular transactions such as withdrawals, bill payments, cheques
- no-fee money orders, certified cheques, traveller's cheques
- discounts on safety deposit boxes.

handle complaints that can't be resolved at the branch. If your parents can't resolve the problem through their bank, there is an independent review process handled by the Ombudsman for Banking Services and Investment (OBSI). Credit unions are provincially regulated and have their own dispute resolution process, so if your parents are clients they can check with them for the correct process of handling complaints.

If your parents have general questions about the Canadian banking system, their rights and the bank's obligations, a quick visit to the Canadian Bankers Association website (www.cba.ca) might help. The CBA has information about banking rules and regulations, safety tips and consumer information booklets.

ELECTRONIC BANKING

Encourage your parents, while they are still actively involved in taking care of their finances, to participate in the world of electronic banking as it will be a huge benefit down the road. As they become less mobile, visits into the bank to deposit cheques and pay bills will not be required. While many people are still reluctant to trust electronic banking, it does offer a safer alternative to your senior parents cashing cheques and paying bills with cash at the bank. If you believe that your parents may balk at this suggestion, you may not be giving them enough credit. Linda's mom was the first in the household to try phone-banking services when they became available and quickly moved on to online banking. Her mom was in charge of paying the household bills and was often the first to discover a new online service. But if your parents are opposed to even trying online banking and you are concerned about their safety, you can arrange to accompany them to the bank.

How we handle our money, pay bills and deal with our investments has changed dramatically in the past decade. While

> Aside from my dad's full-time job, he used to be a treasurer at the church credit union. I remember him going there diligently every Wednesday night. He was always very good when it came to figuring out finances. Over the past few years he has slowly asked my older sister to start helping him with the bills. Looking back now that may have been one of the first signs of him starting to need more help. And he probably was starting to realize that things he used to do so easily were getting harder to do. But for him to remain involved, he would collect up the bills as they came in and file them in a folder. This way when my sister came over regularly to help him sort, review and pay them, it was easy to do.
>
> BARBARA

some seniors still prefer the human contact of dealing with tellers, and receiving their bills in the mail, many more of them have embraced the technological age. It is safe to say that younger seniors today, and the boomer generation following close behind, will be accustomed to online banking.

AUTOMATIC DEPOSIT

Many people now arrange for retirement funds, government cheques and other income to be deposited automatically into their bank account. For your parents, this is safer than receiving payments in the mail and having to visit the bank in person to deposit them. Thieves know when monthly government cheques arrive and they can monitor when an elderly person makes regular visits to the bank. They also can deduce when a senior isn't using the bank and is keeping their money with them or hidden in the house. These situations make seniors prime candidates for robbery. Don't let your parents become victims.

When your parents are no longer as mobile as they were in their younger years, automatic deposits will mean less errands, for them or for you as caregiver. And if your parents are in the hospital for an extended period of time, their funds will still be deposited into their account.

PRE-AUTHORIZED BILL PAYMENTS AND TRANSFERS

Review your parents' list of regular monthly payments and determine if there are expenses that could be set up to be paid automatically from your parents' account. Some examples are payments for car loans, taxes, car insurance, cable, hydro and heating. However, your parents may feel most comfortable having only payments that don't fluctuate set up as pre-authorized payments. If your parents are travelling, have difficulty remembering to pay the bills, or face an extended hospital stay, essential payments will be made without you as caregiver having to step in and do anything.

ELECTRONIC BILL PAYMENT

Almost any company today can be set up to be an online payee, which allows you to pay bills over the phone or on the computer. When regular payments need to be made against an account, you can set up automatic scheduled payouts. If your parents are going to be away for a time, they can even arrange for bills to be paid on a specific date, as one-time payments. Your parents can still receive their statements by mail, or if they are really computer savvy receive them electronically.

If you automate your parents' banking, then you aren't restricted to bank hours when you help them to review their bills and arrange payments. Also, the laborious task of writing cheques and even manually tracking payments in a record book are gone. Statements and account activities are readily available online; you and your parents can easily see what has been paid over several months and identify any missed payments.

If you are at all concerned about the possibility of financial abuse of your aging parents, having bills paid automatically avoids funds sitting in an account, available for someone other than your parents to access.

Accessing Computers

Home computers are becoming increasingly affordable, but for some seniors a home computer, with its monthly provider fee and other maintenance costs, may be outside their budget. If your parents would like to participate in the online world, for pleasure or for personal business, they don't have to own their own computer. Computers are available for public use at many schools, libraries and community centres. If your parents use a public computer for banking purposes, be sure that they are educated about basic online security measures. Another alternative to purchasing a new computer is to buy a used one. Local community centres and senior centres offer computer training courses. Your parents could also come and use your computer if you have one, which would give you an opportunity to visit with them.

Industry Canada supports a program called Community Access Program (CAP), which provides listings of institutions that allow public access to computers and availability of previously owned systems. Here is the website: http://cap.ic.gc.ca/pub/index.html.

Protecting Your Parents' Assets

Seniors are vulnerable to crime, and especially to financial crime. Telemarketing fraud, offering investment opportunities and selling merchandise over the telephone, is one of the most common types of financial crime. Two out of every five victims

TIPS FOR PREVENTING FINANCIAL ABUSE

- Arrange for monthly income to be deposited automatically into accounts (CPP and OAS and any other income they have).
- Arrange to pay as many bills as possible by pre-authorized withdrawal, or via electronic (online) bill payment.
- Set a reasonable daily withdrawal limit at the bank. This prevents someone who has stolen their banking card, or tried to con them from accessing large amounts of money.
- Set reasonable credit card limits, for the same reason.
- Remind your parents never to lend their debit card and PIN number to anyone, not even to family members.
- Seniors are vulnerable when using ATMs and they should be advised not to do so late at night, nor to use ones that are isolated or not well lit.
- Arrange if possible to have credit accounts set up to be paid monthly, on credit cards or through billing. For example, you can arrange an account with a local cab company or companies that deliver meals to the house.

Adapted from Government of Saskatchewan: Justice and Attorney General, "What Families and Friends Can Do Checklist 1: B. Banking and Financial," 2007.

are over the age of sixty years old and 67 percent of them are women.[14] It's hard for most of us to imagine, but it is also not uncommon for family and friends to take advantage of elderly people. There are steps that you can encourage your parents to take to protect themselves from financial abuse.

Preventing Financial Abuse

As caregiver you need to watch for financial abuse, not just by outsiders but from family and friends. It can take many forms,

Financial abuse can involve

- forcing or tricking seniors to sell their home
- stealing or convincing seniors to give/gift money, jewellery, furniture or other belongings
- forging signatures on cheques or other legal documents (perpetrators often find documents to copy in the garbage so encourage your parents to shred important papers)
- forcing or convincing seniors to perform services or lend items without proper compensation, for example, insisting that they look after grand-kids, or using their car, or sharing their home
- misusing power of attorney status.

some of them subtle and involving the misappropriation not only of funds but also belongings.

Someone looking to take advantage of your older parents may threaten and lie, but they may also manipulate them in more sub-tle ways, being friendly and making promises. Generally this type of financial abuse by family and friends is not a one-time occur-rence but takes place over a period of time, making it difficult to identify. Stay in frequent contact with your older parents so that you are aware of who is visiting them, whether any new people have entered their circle of friends, and whether things are miss-ing from their home. Also watch for behavioural changes that would indicate that they are afraid, or being asked to do things that they are not sure about or don't want to do.

As caregiver to your parents you will have to respect their

SIGNS OF FINANCIAL ABUSE[16]

To detect financial abuse, be alert for the following:

- Your parents suddenly have large sums of money being taken out of their bank account.
- They are suddenly in debt and don't know why.
- They have changed or are talking about changing their will.
- Jewellery, clothes and other items are missing from their house.
- Your parents can't remember signing papers, transferring funds or taking money out of the bank, but it has taken place.
- Your parents are slowly isolating themselves from family and friends.
- Your parents seem worried or scared when the subject of money is discussed.

wishes if they don't want to acknowledge and report a situation to the police. However, if you think that your parents have fallen victim to an abuser due to an incapacitated ability and you don't have any other recourse, you can contact the Public Guardian and Trustee, which will investigate and act on your parents' behalf (see the Senior and Caregiver Resource Guide).

Elder abuse, both physical and financial, is a concern of our governments and law enforcement agencies and there are many online resources through which you can obtain information and help if you know of anyone who is a victim.

PhoneBusters is the Canadian anti-fraud call centre that offers information about fraud, tips for prevention and a place to report suspected fraud. Toll-free 1-888-495-8501, www.phonebusters.com.

ROLE OF THE PUBLIC GUARDIAN AND TRUSTEE

The Public Guardian and Trustee is appointed by the Lieutenant Governor in Council and is established under the Public Guardian and Trustee Act. The Office of the Public Guardian and Trustee

- administers the property and finances of adults who are incapable of managing their financial affairs, monitors other property guardians and investigates allegations of financial abuse
- has authority to investigate allegations of financial abuse and to freeze bank accounts under certain circumstances
- administers the estates of deceased persons
- holds and administers unclaimed property
- protects the property rights of children under the age of eighteen.

See our Senior and Caregiver Resource Guide for your province's contact information.

Estate Planning

In Chapter 2, we talked about having conversations with our parents to determine how they had prepared financially for the future, for the time when they can't look after themselves. Estate planning is the process of arranging your affairs so that in the event of your death or mental incapacity your wishes concerning your property and personal care will be carried out by your family. Online forms and packages can be purchased to help you through the steps of creating power of attorney and wills. The process may be complicated, depending on your financial situation, so it's usually best to work with a lawyer to draw up the legal documents. Also, working through a lawyer is another way to prevent your senior parents from being vulnerable to fraud.

The key legal documents that need to be prepared are enduring power of attorney, power of attorney for personal care, and a will. In this section, we review the various types of power of attorney and why it's imperative that your parents have identified power of attorney, and highlight some of the differences that occur between provinces. We also look at why you should ensure your senior parents have a will and what information you need to have ready in the event of your parents' death.

POWER OF ATTORNEY

Much of your time acting as caregiver for your parents will involve your working together to make decisions for them. But there may come a time when your aging parents are no longer competent to act for themselves. A power of attorney is a legal document stating that one person gives another person the full power and authority to represent him or her. But it isn't that simple. The laws pertaining to power of attorney are under provincial jurisdiction, so terms referring to these documents and restrictions vary significantly from province to province. In British Columbia, for example, a power of attorney agreement needs to be registered by the registrar before it can take effect. Who can be granted power of attorney varies in each province, too, with some age and other restrictions. In various provinces the person creating the power of attorney can be called the principle or the grantor, and the person being granted the power, the attorney or agent. No matter what they are called,

> Different types of power of attorney are also given different names, for example, Alberta has an Enduring Power of Attorney and a Personal Directive, British Columbia has a Representation Agreement and a Health Care Directive.

the various powers of attorney are created to provide legal protection for your parents. You will need to research your province's specific rules before working with your parents to establish the required power of attorney.

REGULAR POWER OF ATTORNEY

This basic power of attorney is used often in business, and is established to allow someone to act on another's behalf in financial and legal matters. It can be very general, giving someone wide powers to deal with assets, or it can be specific about what you are allowing them to do for you. For example, if someone was going to be out of the country for a time, they might set up a power of attorney to allow another person to run their business while they were away. Or someone who needed to have a car sold but was unable to take care of it themselves might give someone else power of attorney to manage the sale.

In your role as caregiver a general power of attorney would be useful if your parents were hospitalized for a time and they wanted to assign someone to pay the bills, or cash cheques, or take care of other financial or legal matters. Even if your parents were not hospitalized, a general power of attorney could be set up so that you were able to assist with financial and legal matters on behalf of your parents. Your parents can assign very specific powers to more than one person, the powers can apply to a defined time period, and the power of attorney can be revoked at any time. Your parents should keep in mind that if there is more than one person named as power of attorney matters can become complicated.

Contact your bank and the federal Service Canada offices in your area for forms specifically for setting up a power of attorney for access to bank accounts and to cash federal cheques on your parents' behalf. Check with your banking institution too, as some require you to fill out their own forms even if you've set up a general power of attorney. Be aware that for your parents' protection, banks have restrictions on how they proceed with requests from agents with power of attorney and may require their legal department's approval before they are able to act.

Definition of *incapable* or *lacking capacity*: not being able to understand information that is relevant to decision-making and not being able to evaluate the consequences of making the decision.

One mistake that people make is thinking that once they have set up a power of attorney while they are healthy and capable, they also have plans in place in the event that they suddenly become incapacitated. However, this general power of attorney is based on the principle that someone is capable when making the request and while the powers are being carried out. When your parents become incapacitated, mentally incompetent or die, this type of power of attorney ends.

ENDURING POWER OF ATTORNEY

The different provinces give this various names, but the principle is the same. An enduring power of attorney is prepared when your parents are competent to identify who they want to make decisions concerning their financial and legal affairs in the event that they become mentally incapacitated because of dementia, coma or other means and can no longer make decisions. An enduring power of attorney comes into effect only when it has been determined that your parents are incapable or are lacking the capacity to make decisions.

Within the enduring power of attorney your parents can stipulate *how* they are to be determined incapable; for example, they could name a specific doctor to make the diagnosis, or request a certain number of doctors to sign off on the diagnosis, or even request a mental competency assessment before the person assigned begins acting on their behalf. As well your parents can name more than one person to be their agent.

If your parents receive a diagnosis that would invoke the enduring power of attorney and they feel that it is a mistake and they are still capable, they have recourse. They have a right to request a capacity review hearing and they can hire a lawyer to represent them in court. This is important for you and your parents in the event that you feel someone is forcing the enactment of enduring power of attorney.

If your parents become incapacitated and don't have an enduring power of attorney, there isn't an automatic appointment of spouse or child to take on the responsibility. The immediate family or other relative or friend must apply to the court and request to be appointed. If several people want the role, or contest the person who is applying, the result could be an expensive and lengthy court case. Until that person is appointed, you and your family won't be able to access funds or take care of your parents' other financial obligations. Also, once the court appoints a trustee, it will require a detailed breakdown of all the assets and property and will require periodic accounting of how these are being managed.

If you care for both parents, you should be aware that there are limits on what a spouse is able to manage on their own, especially in terms of jointly owned property. Anything that requires both signatures to be dealt with cannot be managed by one parent.

The general power of attorney and enduring power of attorney will prove invaluable when you and your family need to step in and start helping your aging parents, or if circumstances require you to take over their financial and legal affairs.

I am a certified personal support worker who specializes in dementia and palliative care. Home care is my chosen field. Even my education and experience didn't fully prepare me for the anguish I went through with my own parents when I had to intervene in their lives and take over invoking their powers of attorney for health and property. This took over three years of struggling to get them to accept the help that they desperately needed, but refused to allow. My father was diagnosed with Alzheimer's disease, and my mother had suffered from multiple sclerosis and was almost completely bedridden.

One day my mother had a stroke and fell out of bed. My father could not pick her up. He left her on the floor for quite some time because he did not want to bother the neighbours. My brother had been away for the weekend and called an ambulance when he discovered the situation. My mother refused to go to the hospital and just wanted to be put back into bed. A nurse was directed to their home to follow up on the situation. Mom ended up in the hospital, and I left work to come up and deal with the situation.

Dad could not be left alone in the house. He was too frail and too far along with Alzheimer's to be able to cope without Mom giving him direction. The house insurance company would not cover them with his condition. I managed to plead with his doctor to get him into the geriatric assessment centre. It broke my heart when the doctor asked if I needed the police to come with me. I declined, and tricked Dad into going under the premise that Mom needed him and that he needed to be checked out to make sure it was okay for him to be with her during her stay. I knew that neither one of them was going to be able to go home again. Dad failed his assessment and was malnourished. Mom was hemiplegic and had a pressure sore that went right down to her tailbone from staying in one position.

I was then able to invoke my powers of attorney for Mom because we had had a business meeting about this several years before. I was surprised to discover that Dad also had delegated me as his. I had to get them into long-term care, find their documents, sell their house, and deal with over fifty years of their life together. Many of their bills were over a year in arrears, including their taxes. They could have lost their house. My Dad died this past March after two and a half years in long-term care. My mother is not happy, but she is safe and well cared for. Their years of self-imposed, silent desperation were halted just before the worst-case scenario was realized. It wasn't easy on anyone.

While the right to autonomy is central to protecting people, it can get very precarious when dealing with the frail and elderly.

LESLEY, TORONTO, ONTARIO

POWER OF ATTORNEY FOR PERSONAL CARE

What happens when your parents become incapacitated and need medical care? Different provinces call the power of attorney for personal care by different names, and they have different rules around who can be named to this role and what you can decide on your parents' behalf. In general the power of attorney for personal care allows your parents to name one or more persons to make decisions not only about medical treatments in the hospital, but about their personal care such as nutrition, clothing and personal safety. Again they can be as general as they like, empowering the appointed person to make all personal decisions in their best interest, or they can be specific about what they wish to have happen with regard to medical treatment, housing and general health care. As with enduring power of attorney, your parents can stipulate the circumstances under which you as caregiver, or whoever they name, would begin making personal care decisions on their behalf.

Some people think of a "living will" in terms of specifying their wishes regarding health care, and more specifically, in specifying their wishes about medical treatment and life-sustaining procedures and organ donations in the event that they are unable to express their wishes verbally. Examples are whether they would want to be sustained by medical equipment if in a coma, or under what circumstances they would not want to be resuscitated. In Canadian law we do not have "living wills"; instead a power of attorney for personal care would outline the treatment levels and other related wishes.

To invoke a power of attorney you must present a notarized copy of the document. If you have a power of attorney, either have a copy or know where it is kept.

If your parents become incapacitated without a power of attorney for personal care, the law provides that the family can make decisions about treatments, admission to care facilities

UNDERSTANDING POWER OF ATTORNEY

- Power of attorney (regular): a document that appoints another person to make financial and legal decisions for you. It can be general or specific. It automatically ends if you become bankrupt, die or become mentally incompetent.
- Enduring power of attorney: a document that appoints another person to make financial and legal decisions for you in the event that you become mentally incompetent.
- Power of attorney for personal care: a document that appoints another person to make decisions about your health care and personal

care. It includes your wishes about life-sustaining procedures and treatments, and organ donation.

- A power of attorney is not part of the will and should be kept separate. The power of attorney is only legal when a person is living.
- By having an enduring power of attorney and a power of attorney for personal care, you prevent others stepping in and making decisions on your behalf or on behalf of your family.
- While still mentally competent you can change or revoke your powers of attorney at any time.
- You can appoint more than one person to act as attorney, and you can have separate people acting on your behalf for financial/legal decisions and health/care decisions. Naming more than one person can complicate decision making.
- The persons named in your powers of attorney are not obligated to take on the position, so be sure to talk to those you are choosing to ensure they understand your wishes and agree to accept the responsibility.
- Some provinces require a lawyer to create a power of attorney, and in some provinces you need to register your power of attorney. Some provinces limit the authority you are able to convey if you haven't gone through a lawyer.
- Check your province's laws pertaining to power of attorney; more than just the names are different. The rules for preparation, the scope of authority and types of responsibilities vary by province.

You will find information about power of attorney in your province through the Public Guardian and Trustee contact information in our Senior and Caregiver Resource Guide.

and hospitals, and personal assistance services. The law gives this decision-making authority based on the following hierarchy: spouse/partner, parent/child, sibling, and finally any other relative. Again this varies province by province and involves some degree of governmental involvement and reporting.

By now you will have seen that taking the time to prepare an enduring power of attorney and power of attorney for personal care is important not just for your aging parents, but for yourself as well.

WILLS

All powers of attorney end upon your parents' death and their will takes over to speak for them. The will is likely the document with which you are most familiar and that you are most likely to have had drawn up for yourself. If your parents don't have a will, encourage them to make one.

If your parents die without a will, the government will step in and appoint an administrator for the estate. Usually the spouse or partner is appointed, but if there isn't a spouse/partner or they do not want or cannot perform the responsibility, others can apply for the role: members of the immediate family, relatives, or any other appropriate person, including a friend,

THREE IMPORTANT REASONS TO HAVE A WILL

- To tell family what is to be done with assets or property and personal property.
- To name an executor who will ensure that what is outlined in the will is carried out, including funeral requests and estate management.
- To appoint a guardian if there are children or other dependents.

FINANCIAL AND LEGAL ISSUES

EXECUTORS

Naming an executor is an important decision. Things to consider when making the choice:

- Does this person have good administrative skills?
- Does this person have an understanding of finances and the ability to deal with legal matters?
- Does he/she live close by?
- Is he/she able to and willing to devote the time necessary?

The executor can appoint an administrator to carry out the responsibilities if he/she is unable to or chooses not to.

lawyer or accountant. If no one is suitable, the Public Guardian and Trustee will take on the position.

If your parents die without a will, their assets will be distributed according to provincial legislation. In most cases there is a rule of order in dividing property among the family. Ultimately, in addition to the family arguments and the stress caused by your parents having no will, they will have lost the opportunity to decide who will look after their affairs when they are gone, or to ensure that any important belongings go to particular people.

Your parents don't need a lawyer to draw up a will, but if the estate is significant or complicated it is advisable to work through a lawyer specializing in wills. This ensures that your parents do not experience duress when preparing their will. A lawyer can also help minimize the income taxes and provincial estate administration fees owing when the estate is administered.

August 2006: more unfortunate news for my mum. Lung cancer, terminal this time. She chose not to do chemo as it would have only made her sicker, quicker. Now my siblings and I had to prepare for everything. The majority of the responsibility lay with my brother who was one of the two executors. The support and communication was my responsibility. With everyone all over the world (UK, Alberta and Ontario), thank goodness for conference calling and e-mails.

Mum passed in January 2007. With both parents gone, the estate issues begin. If you have a tight, understanding family things will go smoothly no matter what. I've heard stories of families getting into wars over estates. Thankfully not with ours. My brother took care of that, though he did say it can be overwhelming when you are getting different information from lawyers and accountants. The more information and understanding you have about the estate, the better you will be prepared.

SHEILA, GRIMSBY, ONTARIO

The purpose of this section was not to advise you or your parents on how to draw up a will but to highlight the importance of having your parents' legal and financial areas in order as they advance through the stages of aging. If they haven't done this, as they get on in years and possibly end up no longer mentally capable of drawing up a will, or setting up enduring powers of attorney or powers of attorney for personal care, you and your family will be left scrambling at a time when you also have your parents' care to worry about.

Planning Ahead for Funerals

The executor is the only person with the legal authority to "control the disposition" for the deceased. In other words, he or she is the only one allowed to make the funeral arrangements. If your parents want someone specific, other than the named executor of your will, to take on this special task, they must put it into their will.

Be aware that funeral homes and cemeteries are prohibited from direct-selling at a person's residence unless your parents have invited them. To protect your parents' interest, the funeral home representative is required to set the appointment after a twenty-four-hour waiting period. This is important to know in the event that your parents are talking about being visited by someone trying to sell them funeral services or plots.

PREPAID/PLANNED FUNERAL ARRANGEMENTS

Your parents can plan a funeral without paying for anything, either on their own or in conjunction with a funeral home. The plans stay on file, at home or at the funeral home, so that when the time comes, the family knows what he or she wanted.

If they prepay for their funeral, the money is put into a government-regulated trust account. The rules around these vary across the provinces, so do some research. For example, money paid for a prepaid funeral in B.C. has to be put into a trust account within twenty-one days, while in Ontario it's ten days. And in Ontario the funeral home is required to send proof through annual account statements of where and how the money was invested. A prepaid agreement may be cancelled at any time; again, check your provincial rules, as in some provinces the funeral provider is entitled to keep a percentage of the amount received for selling expenses. In British Columbia it's 20 percent of the amount received, while in Ontario it's 10 percent and only up to a maximum of two hundred dollars.

If a funeral is prepaid and the funeral doesn't take place for several years, the amount charged does not increase even if over the years the costs of those services have. But keep in mind that this rule varies depending on whether your parents have paid for the funeral in full, or are paying for it by the month. Again, check the rules in your province and read the fine print of the contract before your parents sign anything.

There are lots of books and websites out there to help you explore the subject of funeral planning. It is important to communicate with your parents and plan ahead in order to make this emotional time a bit easier to navigate. Even if they don't want to plan their funeral ahead, you can find out through discussion what your parents want. It's a difficult subject, but as your parents get older, you may find that they want to talk about the past, and also about what they are facing. Approach the subject with sensitivity and maybe even humour.

Upon a Parent's Death

When your parents pass away, you will need specific information right away, and you should know where to find it. On the facing page is a list of the information that the executor of the estate may require.

Your parents should have key legal matters in place before

A BOOK FOR GRIEVING

Tear Soup: A Recipe for Healing After Loss is a family story book that emphasizes the individual nature of grief through the making of soup. The main character, Grandy, has just suffered a big loss in her life, and so she begins to make her "tear soup." *Tear Soup* is a wonderful book for anyone who has experienced a loss. By Pat Schwiebert and Chuck DeKlyen and illustrated by Taylor Bills (Grief Watch, 1999).

KEY INFORMATION REQUIRED

You will need the following upon your parents' death:

Personal information:

- [ ] SIN
- [ ] dates and places of parents' birth
- [ ] your grandparents' names and places of birth
- [ ] military service number
- [ ] proof of citizenship
- [ ] telephone number

Documents:

- [ ] will
- [ ] birth certificate
- [ ] marriage licence
- [ ] insurance documents (health, life, car, house, accident)
- [ ] property deeds
- [ ] auto ownership
- [ ] income tax returns
- [ ] military discharge papers

the aging process takes away their ability to make decisions. As a family member you can lead by example; have your own legal documents prepared and ensure that your parents know where you have put them in the event that you are involved in an accident or face a medical crisis.

We have reviewed many serious issues and life-altering scenarios that as a caregiver you will be involved in with your parents.

Likely you have recognized that the role you have taken on will be a major part of your life going into the future. Finding ways to manage and take care of yourself will be critical for you to be successful in this role. In the next chapter we focus on you, as caregiver.

My mom made me executor of her estate. In some ways I wasn't the best choice for the job—I don't really have a head for numbers and I don't know much about dealing with lawyers and mortgage agents—but there really wasn't anyone else for my mom to choose.

I couldn't imagine being the executor for someone with a really complicated estate. The amount of time involved, the different dealings with banks, lawyers, creditors, utilities was very stressful, especially when I was still recovering from the loss. I initially took a week off work to make all the phone calls to notify all the necessary people, and to write letters to accompany the death certificates that I had to send out. Luckily, I had good administrative skills so keeping track of the paperwork wasn't an issue.

I think the hardest part was making the actual calls. Call after call, telling people that my mom was dead and I was the executor. Everyone I spoke with was very nice and knew exactly what needed to be done, but at the end of each day my sadness was more than I could bear. Months later there still seemed to be so much to do and I didn't really feel I could rest and truly grieve until all the legal matters of the estate were finalized.

The job of executor requires someone who is organized, has the time, and some business sense. While it is logical to pick a family member, if the estate is large and complicated with property, investments, lots of heirs, then choose the executor carefully. There is a lot of responsibility and many things to do during a very emotional time.

LINDA

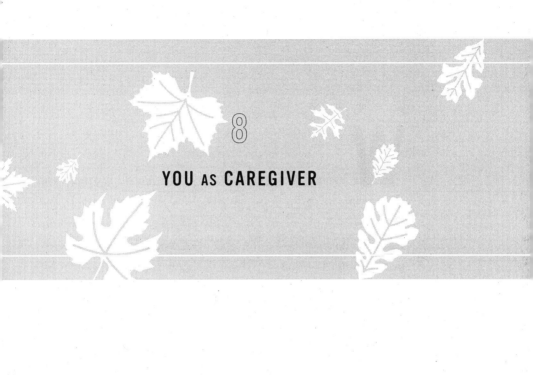

8

YOU AS CAREGIVER

We have talked about many of the issues you may encounter in caring for your parents. Now let's focus on you, the caregiver. You are managing many responsibilities, personally and probably professionally, and balancing the needs of many people. You may wonder where the time you used to have for yourself has gone. It's not uncommon to experience feelings of anger, guilt, frustration, stress, worry and doubt. You are making important decisions, dealing with family personalities, managing limited amounts of time, manoeuvreing through administrative red tape, taking care of your family and continuing to work. You are also trying to come to terms with the fact that your parents are in need and may be in pain, and may even be coming to the end of their lives.

If you are to be successful as a caregiver in safeguarding your parents' health, you must look after yourself mentally and physically. Strive for a balance between your role as a caregiver and the other roles in your life. In this chapter we'll talk about

- how being a caregiver develops your personal skills
- how the stress of caregiving can affect your health
- how good time management skills can help you and your family

- how to balance home, work and caregiving responsibilities
- support options through work and government assistance
- ways you can look after yourself
- the importance of fostering personal support systems
- the role of respite care.

Being the Caregiver

Being the caregiver for your aging parents requires not only your time but also the ability to develop new skills and draw on skills that you may already use in your job or family life. You need to be able to plan ahead, manage your time, and identify and assemble information to accomplish tasks. How much support you receive in your role as caregiver can greatly affect how you feel about the responsibilities. If you're getting practical assistance and emotional encouragement from family and/or the community, you will perceive your role as caregiver in a more positive way.

Your reasons for having taken on the role also affect the type of caregiver you are and how you will perceive the tasks you perform for your parents. For many of us our feelings of love for our parents and the knowledge that they sacrificed for us gives us a sense of responsibility for our parents. We make the choice, even if unconsciously in the early stages, because of everything we feel our parents have given us throughout our lives. But some adult children do not have a strong relationship with their parents and do the caregiving out of a sense of guilt and obligation. Regardless of your reason for taking on this important task, you need to look after yourself in order to care for your parents.

Dealing with Stress

We encounter varying degrees of stress throughout our lives, and being able to identify it is the start to understanding what

Two years ago, my mother began to slip away from me. She was diagnosed with a form of dementia called Lewy body disease and although she remained relatively symptom free at first, it wasn't long before her mind began to deteriorate and it soon became obvious that she would need full-time care. Unwilling to face this fact, I took a year off of work and became my mother's primary caregiver. All of this occurred just after my thirty-seventh birthday—an age when I was officially an adult, yet still felt young enough that the task of caring for my mother seemed somewhat unreal.

I am the youngest of five children and my mother had me very late in life. Growing up, she was the oldest of all my friends' mothers, and even now, she is somewhat of a wonder among my friends, as most women find the thought of having a fifth child at the age of forty to be quite daunting. I often teased my mother about her decision to have me, alluding to the fact that I must have been a mistake. She would smile and tell me that there was always room at the table for another mouth to feed. And then she would inevitably change the topic.

There were many days, and still are, when I curse the fates and question how such a terrible disease could happen to such a good woman. Where is the justice? Why had this happened to our family? But these self-pitying questions soon took a back seat to the task at hand: caring for my rapidly declining mother.

For the past two years, I have watched as my mother's mind has deteriorated into a world of paranoia and hallucinations. And as the dementia destroyed her mentally, she suffered physically as well.

Cooking her meals eventually evolved into cutting her food, and at times feeding her. Helping her in and out of the shower eventually became a full-body wash that would end with wrapping her in a towel and drying her off as she had done to me so many years ago. Sorting her laundry became dressing her in the morning and undressing her at night. Sitting by her side in comfortable silence became sitting by her bed, holding her hand as she suffered through another illness brought on by a change in medication.

One day, toward the end of my time as her caregiver at home, as her mind descended into a madness that I could not alleviate, I tried to pull her back to reality with my age-old teasing of how a fifth child at the age of forty must have been a mistake.

And to my surprise and joy, she looked at me with clear eyes, free of the uncertainty and fear that usually clouded them, and she said, "People thought I was foolish for having a child so late in life. But I look at you and thank God that I did because you take such good care of me now."

Sadly, it is through my mother's dementia that I have gained a sense of clarity. I would bargain with the Devil if I could reverse her disease. But knowing that I can't, I have found the last few years to be the most challenging in my life and the most fulfilling. I have given back to a woman who gave up more for me than I could possibly ever imagine. I have learned what it truly means to love and respect another human being. I have grown closer to the rest of my family as we all step up to support and protect the matriarch who defined our lives.

And I have laughed with my mother and cried with my mother, but most of all, I have been there for her as she was for me as I was growing up.

DIANE, TORONTO, ONTARIO

we need to do to get through it. Stress is not only mentally draining but can result in physical symptoms as well, manifesting itself as headache, upset stomach, disrupted sleep, anger at others, confusion and anxiety. Stress can also make it harder for you to fight off disease, because it lowers your immune system.

I am the sole caregiver of my disabled, senior father who is now seventy-eight years of age. I have been his sole caregiver now for over fifteen years. It has been very difficult for me. I have not been able to work for the past two years as he is too ill to live alone any more. My father refuses to go into a home and we agreed he would die at home. This decision was made long before he became very ill and it has been a difficult one for me to stand by. I do receive home care but only to shower him and change his disposable diapers. I am responsible for all his care, financial and otherwise. I am his legal guardian. This has affected my life in many ways. I am forty-three years old now and have literally no life. I am confined to my home and am as isolated from the world as he is. I could never believe it would be this heart-wrenching. To sit and watch someone die on a daily basis takes so much out of a person.

My youngest daughter has been a lifesaver for me. She is twenty-two and has given up so much of her life for him, and it hurts me to see her suffer as she does. She loves her grandpa but it is so hard for her also. He is very needy and takes so much time and energy. It drains the life out of us. It is very difficult to care for an elderly parent but it is something I would never give up because when he is gone, he is gone and then there is no more. Life is not fair but no one said it would be.

BRENDA, EDMONTON, ALBERTA

And it can drain your energy. Whether the tasks you face are small, like picking up a prescription for your parents during a hectic day, or large, like previewing long-term care facilities, as a caregiver you should learn to identify the signs of stress.

Self-awareness is important. Trust yourself and your abilities. Know yourself and your reactions so that you can recognize when you are reaching your limit. Acknowledge the feelings that you are having as you look after your parents. Don't put off making decisions as this can increase stress. And don't put off doing tasks, as they will be on your mind until they are completed. Delegate tasks to others whenever possible but especially when you need to take a break. Use your time management skills to balance the responsibilities of caregiving with the responsibilities of your life.

Time Management

Good time management skills will help reduce stress and allow you to find some time for yourself.

Realistically, there will be times when your parents will require urgent attention and their needs cannot be dictated by a schedule. Sometimes you will feel there is not enough time in the day to get your parents everything they need. Or you will feel that things seem not to move fast enough. Recognizing that you can't always control your time can help reduce stress.

TIME MANAGEMENT TIPS

- Keep a calendar that combines your appointments with those of your parents.
- Maintain a to-do list and prioritize items.
- Streamline your finances. Pay bills by automatic withdrawal or use online banking.
- Hold regular meetings of the immediate family to delegate tasks.
- Combine errands to save time.
- Designate a family communication centre, where you keep phone messages, the family calendar and special instructions.

- Be clear with instructions and leave written notes if required.
- Create a list of days and times when extended family are available to help, so that you can schedule tasks for them too.
- Develop effective communication systems within your extended family (e.g., a phone tree, group e-mails).
- Prepare for each day the night before (lay out clothes, gather paperwork, know the day's schedule).
- Book time for yourself in order to avoid burnout and to give yourself something to look forward to.

Balancing Caregiving and Your Home Life

When you take on the responsibility of being a caregiver for your parents, you do not give up all the other responsibilities in your life. Trying to balance caregiving for aging parents with family and home obligations can be a significant cause of stress. When you overextend yourself trying to manage everything, you feel that you're not taking care of anything properly. Recognizing that you can't do it all, and finding other solutions to getting things done will lessen the burden.

FAMILY MEALS

Ensuring everyone in the house is getting fed can be a challenge if you have to be with your parents for long periods of time or if you need to be with them during mealtimes. This can cause feelings of guilt because you are not at home caring for your family. Completing caregiving tasks may make it difficult for you to get your own errands, such as grocery shopping, done. Sharing tasks and establishing routines will lessen your responsibilities and reduce your stress.

TIPS FOR MEAL PREPARATION

- Prepare meals for the week in advance and freeze.
- Try commercially prepared frozen meals.
- Find out if there are companies in your area that offer fresh, prepared meals requiring limited cooking time.
- Have a running grocery list posted to which everyone in the household can add items.
- Order groceries online.
- Ask other family members to help with shopping and meal preparation.
- Combine shopping trips with your parents' errands.
- Have older children do the grocery shopping.
- Encourage kids to help make meals for the family or selves.
- Order takeout periodically.
- Talk with partner about taking on more cooking responsibility.

When in crisis

- Have a service such as Meals on Wheels deliver to your home.
- Arrange for children to eat at a friend's or neighbour's house.

HOUSEWORK

Maintaining a house is also stressful. You have to learn to let go of some of the expectations that things need to be perfect. Prioritize the housework and decide where to focus your energy. Don't feel guilty if you decide to hire outside help.

Balancing Caregiving and Work Life

Another difficult aspect of caregiving is trying to keep up with the demands of your job, especially when caregiving in itself

> Throughout all the frustration, lost wages for missing work, all the tears I cry that no one will ever see, there will come a day that I will be able to look back and be thankful that I had this time to spend with them. I will never look back and wish I would have done this, or taken them there. I have done everything for them that I can. There will be no regrets. I think there may be for other family members, but that will be their cross to bear.
>
> They gave me the best child-hood and life they could, and I'm sure I wasn't always the greatest child to have, and I've heard that what goes around, comes around, so now it's my turn to help them when they are weak and I am the stronger one.
>
> It's called unconditional love.
>
> LORI, KITCHENER, ONTARIO

seems to be a full-time job! Depending on the stage of care you are at with your parents, you can investigate various workplace options to reduce the pressure. Only you can determine at what point you should have a discussion with your supervisor about your situation. If you're lucky, you have a work environment that can accommodate your situation so that you don't need to take extended leave time until your parents require you full time.

You may also want to take the opportunity to let your supervisor know how much information about your circumstances you would like them to share with your co-workers and how much should remain confidential.

An increasing number of companies are recognizing that outside stresses have an impact on an employee's ability to work productively. As the caregiving community grows, companies should acknowledge the need for change in the workplace to accommodate their employees who are also caregivers to aging parents. Over the past few years, many workplaces have adapted to employees with children; similarly, employers should take into consideration the needs of employees who are caregivers to the elderly.

Government Assistance

When the time comes that your parents require intensive care, you may want to consider taking an extended leave from work.

Check with your supervisor or your human resource department to see if you have any benefits available to you through your company. You can also take a compassionate care leave that is offered through the federal government under the Employment Standards Act. It allows you to take a maximum of six weeks off work to provide care for a gravely ill family member. You can get more details and find out how to apply through the Services Canada website (see our Senior and Caregiver Resource Guide for contact information).

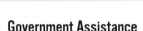 Just weeks prior to my mother-in-law Kay's passing in April 2007, my doctor put me on extended medical leave due to stress, depression and the physical toll it was taking on my body. However, as I sat on with my sister-in-law and we watched Kay take her last breath, I didn't have any regrets about doing everything in my power to take care of a wonderful lady.

JANET, NANAIMO,
BRITISH COLUMBIA

Employment standards vary across provinces so check with your provincial government or talk to human resources at your workplace. For example, in Ontario a family medical leave covers up to eight weeks' job-protected leave for the purpose of attending to a loved one who has become gravely ill or is dying. This leave is available even if you apply for federal compassionate care benefits. Manitoba also offers a family leave of up to eight weeks within a twenty-six-week period.

Another option is to find out whether you're eligible for any tax deductions due to your caregiver status. If you check the Canada Revenue Agency, you may find that you qualify for income tax benefits as a caregiver.

Caring for the Caregiver

No matter how busy you are, schedule time to look after yourself. Remember to nourish your body and spirit. Don't disregard the physical toll that caregiving takes on your body. By making time to look after your own physical health you will find the strength to carry on, and will be in a better frame of mind to deal with the challenges.

EAT PROPERLY

As caregivers we are often so involved in looking after others that we forget to eat. This is especially true during times of crisis. Try to start the day with a good breakfast. Time goes by quickly, so be conscious of your body when it tells you you're hungry. Get in the habit of carrying snacks and water with you. Choose healthy foods to help sustain your energy.

SLEEP WELL

Make sure you get enough sleep, which will strengthen your immune system and help you to think clearly in order to make wise decisions. Develop good sleep habits. Try to keep a regular bedtime and develop a relaxing bedtime routine. By identifying this time for yourself, you prepare your body for rest and quiet your mind for sleep.

EXERCISE

Exercise helps re-energize your body and makes you feel that you can do more. It can help you prepare for the day, or help you relax in the evening. If you're not used to exercise, sign up for a class to get you motivated. This will also prompt you to take time for yourself. Check at your workplace to see if they have lunchtime fitness programs or physical fitness reimbursement benefits. Exercise will give you a sense of self-confidence and accomplishment that will carry through to your caregiving.

FIND WAYS TO RELAX

Relaxing can help you refocus. It can dissolve feelings of anger and frustration and allow you to come back to a problem with a fresh outlook. It can also provide you with time to decompress. Developing techniques to relax doesn't necessarily require large amounts of time away from your responsibilities. Relaxing can be as simple as escaping to a bath with a good book, doing breathing exercises, or practising a hobby you enjoy. You can also attend classes to learn relaxation techniques or meditation. And check with your workplace to see if you are covered for therapeutic massages.

NOURISH YOUR SPIRIT

Just as your body needs nourishing, so do your mind and spirit. Opening your spirit to feelings of hope and renewal allows you to feel replenished. Spend time with family and friends; it will give you the opportunity to focus on something other than your parents. Don't hold in your feelings—confide in a friend or family member who can provide emotional support. Actively adopt a more positive outlook by reading books with encouraging messages, listening to uplifting music or looking for humour in daily events. Laughter can help you get through the difficult times. Do something you enjoy even if it's just a couple of minutes in the day. Focus on the present, as it's easy to start worrying about the future and questioning past decisions.

BE CONFIDENT

Caregiving involves many decisions, from small ones such as grocery shopping to larger ones such as where your parents should live. It's easy to second-guess yourself and to struggle with these decisions. During these times remind yourself that you know your parents better than strangers. If your parents have given you power of attorney, they have faith and trust in your ability to makes decisions for them.

Try not to take the reactions of your parents personally during stressful times, especially if their behaviours are related to an illness, or because they are simply not feeling like themselves. Recognize that your parents' anger or other negative reactions may be a result of fear and confusion. Have empathy for them.

AVOID BURNOUT

Looking after your parents over an extended period of time can be physically and emotionally draining. As a caregiver you may feel that your life is no longer your own and be overwhelmed by the responsibility. If you are feeling angry all the time, alone and isolated, and experiencing moments of anxiety and fear, you might be reaching the burnout stage. If these feelings are severe you may want to seek professional counselling, but there are also many small ways in which you can avoid burnout.

WAYS TO AVOID BURNOUT

- Identify signs of stress early, before they become serious (sleep difficulties, headaches, anger and anxiety).
- Don't suppress your feelings; find a confidant.
- Set realistic goals in order to manage your responsibilities.
- Set aside time for yourself, even if it's only an hour or so per day.
- Join a caregiver support group to share your feelings, and obtain tips and advice, resources, coping tools and useful contacts.
- Don't be afraid to talk about your role as caregiver to friends and colleagues.
- Take advantage of respite care, either formal or through family members.
- Do not feel guilty when you can't do everything.
- If your feelings are severe, talk to a professional counsellor, social worker or psychologist.

FIND SUPPORT

As a caregiver you should have a support system in place. You need to know that you have people you can rely on to help you get through the difficult times and decisions. Don't isolate yourself. Maintain relationships with family and friends, and make an effort to keep up with your network of friends who are not directly involved in the situation. These friends can give you some relief and can listen without judgment. Others more distant from the experience may also provide different perspectives on what you are going through.

There are also various types of support, including one-on-one counselling, group counselling, workshops and seminars.

> They say that there is always one person that patients seem to take all their frustration, anger and rejection out on. That person was me! Before Dad got really ill with cancer, he took me aside and said, "Nancy, if I should ever yell at you, or say something that may hurt you, please disregard it. It will not be me speaking, but the pain I am enduring. I love you!" Those words are what kept me going, kept my tears at bay, and kept my strength up, when I felt so depressed.
>
> NANCY, CALEDON, ONTARIO

These may be offered through community centres, not-for-profit societies and religious groups in your area. There are also Web-based support networks. These groups discuss topics specifically related to caregiving. You can contact them individually to determine what they offer and which would be best for you.

ARRANGE RESPITE CARE

Sometimes as a caregiver you need a structured and scheduled break away from your parents. Feelings such as anger and frustration will only increase if you are exhausted and don't take time to recharge. You will need to acknowledge when you need this relief. Do not feel guilty when taking some time for yourself.

Respite care is provided when someone else takes on the caregiver role so that you can take time away from your parents. This care may be provided by family and friends, or more formally by agencies and facilities. You may need to have someone take on your role temporarily for short time periods, a couple of hours a day, or, if you are going on a vacation, for an extended period.

Various support agencies offer respite care, including the Canadian Red Cross and the Victoria Order of Nurses. These agencies can send someone into your home to give you a break. You can also look into senior day programs for your parents.

Respite care is also offered through retirement homes and long-term care homes, depending on your parents' required level of care. Your parents can stay for short or extended periods of time. Some homes have rooms that are specifically allocated for respite care, where your parents can stay for a short time while you are away or just to give you a break. There is a fee and the rate is usually different than the regular accommodation rate. The facility can provide further information about the types of care offered and the fees.

When you cannot physically and/or emotionally provide further care for your parents, you may have to turn the caregiving role over to another member of the family. You may even need to allow professionals to step in and take over the responsibilities. If this occurs, you may experience feelings of guilt and sadness, but even if you are no longer the primary caregiver for your parents, there are still opportunities for you to remain involved.

> My friend Dorothy was a godsend. I could call her and she would be there to help, even if it was just doing the laundry or vacuuming. Housework was the last on my list, because being there for my mother was my priority. My husband was very patient and my daughter was a typical teenager with more responsibility than normal.
>
> KIM, MAPLE RIDGE, BRITISH COLUMBIA

> Soon the leaves would unfold, washing the landscape with delicate green brushstrokes. Already the forsythia was in bloom, bright yellow beside the remaining patches of snow. But I was too harried to truly enjoy the beauty of that quiet spring morning. It was Sunday and I needed to finish getting Mom ready for church.
>
> Mother was nearly eighty-four, no longer able to manage on her own. Earlier, I had helped her shower, shampoo and dress. I'd then rolled a menagerie of curlers into her hair. Now, I guided her frail body toward the vanity for makeup and a comb-out.

"My foot hurts," she said, limping. Seating Mom in front of the mirror, I began unwinding the rollers.

"Um … toenails … need to be.…" I knew she was searching for the word *clipped*. I didn't comment, hoping she would forget about her feet. I wasn't feeling well. I just wasn't up to dealing with toenails. Besides, there was hardly time to finish getting her ready for church as it was.

I examined Mom's reflection in the mirror. Her white hair looked neatly coiffed and the rouge on her cheeks helped her look more pert. But my heart tugged. Oh, Mama! It wasn't the face I knew. Time had ravaged mother's body and mind. Her face was so thin and deeply lined, her cheeks so hollow. And her eyes … I turned away from the reflection of her sunken eyes—eyes searching to remember.

I bent and kissed Mom's forehead. "You look mighty spiffy," I said, hiding my grief as I assisted her to get up.

"Oooh," she cried after one step.

I helped Mom hobble to a nearby chair. Slipping off her shoes, I then struggled to remove the pair of hose I'd struggled to put on minutes earlier. Mom's toenails were badly neglected.

Gathering scissors, a pair of clippers, a towel and a pan of hot water, I returned and knelt down. With an exhausted sigh, I brushed back my hair. I really didn't need this! What I needed was to go lie down and rest. I'd been ill for a number of years and wasn't feeling well enough to attend church myself! I placed Mom's feet in the water.

Now, I lifted out one foot and began the unpleasant job. Mom's feet were tender and she winced as I struggled with each misshapen nail. Resentment flooded in. Why wasn't someone else doing this? Since Dad's death, my husband and I had sole care of my mother. *Clip*. Well, it wasn't fair. It was about time my siblings took some responsibility and helped out. *Clip*. The burden fell totally on me and I was tired of it. I was being taken advantage of. Here I was the one with a serious health problem, yet I was shouldering all the stress and anxiety of Mom's deteriorating physical and mental health. *Clip.*

Anger and self-pity built, even though I was the only child who lived in the same city as my mother—the only one close enough to be caregiver! My siblings lived miles away and stewardship for Mom had naturally fallen upon me. Straightening up I rubbed my back, took another deep breath, [and] then with distaste tackled another toe.

My resentment crept toward Mother—sweet, blameless Mother. I was appalled at my unwelcomed, atypical feelings. They weren't reasonable or justified—they just were. My, I was in a wonderful Sabbath mood, wasn't I? Finished with one foot, I removed Mom's other foot from the pan and set it dripping upon the towel atop my lap. With the towel ends, I began wiping it dry.

Suddenly my mind flashed to an ancient scene, and to another kneeling upon the floor, washing and drying feet. My eyes welled with tears as the emotion of that biblical image surged through me. I was awed by the intensity of it and the instantaneous change that took place within me. All rancour dissolved. I was filled with reverence and gratitude. And more deeply than ever I was moved by the love I felt for my mother. Tenderly I positioned her foot upon my lap and, blinking to clear my vision, I humbly began work upon another nail.

By that simple, menial task I was powerfully reminded of the privilege and opportunity of service and what a server receives in return. Past the window, a bird flew upward against the sky and with it a poignant question came to mind: how many more springs would I have my dear mother a part of my life?

CAREGIVER, SANDY, UTAH

CONCLUSION

THE REWARDS of CAREGIVING

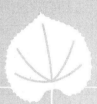

One can easily become overwhelmed at the thought of the negative aspects of caregiving. After all, the responsibilities involved in the role affect so many facets of your life. But there are rewards as well, especially if you focus on the reason you stay involved day in and day out—you are caring for someone you love. Through caregiving you will create a stronger relationship with your parents and gain a different perspective on your life and theirs.

Maintaining a positive outlook will give you a sense of accomplishment and fulfillment. Skills you develop through caregiving, such as communication and time management, can carry through to other aspects of your life. Caregiving increases your ability to care and empathize with others around you. And most of all caregiving can help you to create precious and lasting memories of your parents. When your role as caregiver is over you will have the personal satisfaction of knowing that you helped to give back to your mother and father when it was your turn to parent.

Your parents are on their life's journey and as their caregiver you see their journey as yours. The struggles that come with caregiving are part of the bigger picture of life. And despite those struggles, when asked later most caregivers say that they would choose to do it all again. We have seen this over and over in the

The last couple of years have not been easy. As I started university and eventually moved out of the house, the signs of aging and the issues that come along with it were starting to become more obvious—especially with Dad. I saw my parents starting to move slower, struggling to do things that once were easy, turning to us for more help and forgetting things, and I wondered where the time went. And now I have a greater appreciation for all those family trips to the cottage and the weekend baseball games.

Trying to come to terms with the fact that one day they will not be here to encourage and support me is difficult. I don't think I will ever fully be prepared for that day and so I am grateful for today. I have more patience when I have to run errands and help them out. Enjoying the time that I spend with them now is so important and I make a conscious effort to try to do that. These are the memories I will carry with me for the rest of my life. And I will know that I helped to care for them just as they helped care for me. They mean the world to me and I love them both dearly.

BARBARA

people and the stories throughout this book. Many of the caregivers who contributed to *Our Turn to Parent* reminded us how important it is not to speed through life wishing for another present, and how helping others shows us what really matters in life.

Plan for Your Future

Now that you have read this book about taking care of aging parents, we hope you will also take some time to plan for your own senior years. This book is not only a guide for you as caregiver but a call to action for your own life. The issues in these chapters will become more and more relevant to you as you age.

> When I was young my mom was there for me, and then there were years when we were more friends than child and parent, and eventually I had the chance to be there for her. It's a circle, or perhaps as my mom has said, it's a pattern of life. At first we are close, parent taking care of child, and then we grow apart and lead separate lives, and as both age we come back together but with the child taking on the role of parent, or caregiver, to their parent.
>
> In writing this book I was reminded of a saying that has passed through the generations in our family. My mom repeated this saying to me often, when I walked too fast and looked back to see what was keeping her, or when I had to repeat what I'd said, with a sigh, or when I'd forgotten that my mom needed a coffee break on our errand-running days. It was said by my Nana, my great-grandmother, to her five daughters, including my Auntie Mickie, who was like a grandmother to me, and now by my mother to me—I can hear all their voices in my head. . . .
>
> "Someday you will be old."
>
> I always tried to remember without having to be told.
>
> LINDA

Recognize that you need to plan ahead. Make the financial plans you need to continue the lifestyle you want to live. Think about where you wish to live as you grow older. Make sure that your legal documents are up to date. Think about who you want to be *your* caregiver. The more plans you have in place, the less work there will be for whoever is helping you.

For now, the role of caregiver is yours. We hope you will find in *Our Turn to Parent* some of the tools to get you started and that your experience of caring for your aging parents will be a rewarding one.

ACKNOWLEDGMENTS

We would like to thank everyone at Random House of Canada for their support, especially Anne Collins and Marion Garner for believing that we could write *Our Turn to Parent,* our editor Kendall Anderson for helping us find the right words, and Kelly Hill for creating a wonderful design for our book.

We extend our gratitude to all the caregivers who shared their stories with us. They give the book its heart.

Our appreciation goes to David Grad, Betty Heininger, Grant Moyle, Craig Parker and Pat Schneider for their guidance and enthusiasm.

Barbara would like to thank her family and friends who have always supported and encouraged her, especially Bernadette, Joan, Doug, Dan, Aidan and Sarah.

Linda would like to thank her husband, David, for his love and encouragement over the years and her family, Philip, Linda, Daniel and Ken, for their love and support.

And special thanks to our parents, Bill and Eileen Dunn and Dorene Scott, who are the inspiration for *Our Turn to Parent* and who have encouraged us throughout our lives.

SENIOR AND CAREGIVER
RESOURCE GUIDE

How to Use This Guide

In this guide you will find resources to help seniors and care-givers. Many of the contacts that we have mentioned through-out the book are listed here, including programs for seniors, support organizations for caregivers, social service agencies we have mentioned in the text, good caregiver websites, provincial health organizations, ministry of justice and health departments for each province and many more.

The guide begins with national resources and then is organized by province.

Some listings have a brief description of what you'll find on a website or what you can contact the organization about. Certain provinces have excellent general caregiving sites, so if you don't find helpful information in your own province you could browse other province's websites.

Some province's websites have a "Seniors' Guide" that contains a comprehensive listing of services available within the province. It contains valuable information and is a good starting point for research. Where available they are indicated.

The term "Social Services Support and Assessment" has been used to refer to the government agency that will assign a case manager to assess your parents' care needs. This person develops a care plan, coordinates support services, provides housing options (assisted living and long-term care), determines eligibility for services and funding.

NATIONAL RESOURCES
FEDERAL GOVERNMENT RESOURCES

Canada Benefits
Service Canada
Toll-free: 1-800-622-6232
Website: www.canadabenefits.gc.ca
What you'll find here:
- I Am a Senior section
- information on retirement, health concerns, tax, housing and home modifications, dealing with death, and compassionate care benefits; forms and links
- searchable list of information by province

Canada Revenue Agency
Website: www.cra.gc.ca
What you'll find here:
- guides, forms and publications about federal programs, including ones for seniors; information about what to do following a death, and tips for general security and reporting fraud
- searchable list of information by province

Community Access Program
Industry Canada
Website: http://cap.ic.gc.ca/pub/index.html

What you'll find here:

- information on how to find and access computers

Health Canada

E-mail: info@hc-sc.gc.ca

Website: www.hc-sc.gc.ca

What you'll find here:

- senior information for healthy living, Just for You—Seniors section and listing by topic; information about injury prevention, physical activity, seniors and aging, vision care, falls in the home, end-of-life care, assistive devices, mental health; forms and links
- regional office contact information, which can also be found in the government pages of your phone book

Public Health Agency of Canada

130 Colonnade Road

A.L. 6501H

Ottawa, ON K1A 0K9

1015 Arlington Street

Winnipeg, MB R3E 3R2

Website: www.phac-aspc.gc.ca

What you'll find here:

- general information about senior health, health promotion, assistive devices, caring for seniors, palliative care, injury prevention, seniors accessing computers, medication, *Canada's Physical Activity Guide to Healthy Active Living for Older Adults*, and links.
- online forms for e-mail inquiries
- regional office contact information

Seniors Canada

Website: www.seniors.gc.ca

What you'll find here:

- general information and services for seniors across Canada
- information about caregiving (associations, resources and respite care), housing, end of life, finances and pensions, health and wellness, legal matters, retirement, safety and security, senior networks, travel and leisure; link to the RCMP website, which has the *Seniors' Guidebook to Safety and Security*
- links to major government and provincial websites
- searchable database of information, by province and topic

Service Canada

Canada Enquiry Centre

Ottawa, ON K1A 0J9

Toll-free: 1-800-622-6232

Website: www.servicecanada.gc.ca

What you'll find here:

- *Services for Seniors Guide* (call to order a copy of the guide, or visit a Service Canada Centre)
- senior section with an A-to-Z list of topics, including retirement planning, home adaptation for seniors, housing programs, income assistance, legal assistance such as victim services, personal documents such as Old Age Security ID, savings plans information
- caregiver section that includes links to information on caregiver amount for tax returns, taking care of yourself, exploring live-in caregiver options (under Families and Children)
- Employment Insurance compassionate care leave information:

  www.servicecanada.gc.ca/en/sc/ei/benefits/compassionate.shtml

All Canadian Pet Services Network

P.O. Box 72551

345 Bloor Street East Unit #5

Toronto, ON M4W 3S9

Website: www.acpsn.com

What you'll find here:

- a national not-for-profit support organization for petsitters and dog walkers
- pet service providers who offer respite care are listed with contact information

Alzheimer Society of Canada

20 Eglinton Avenue West, Suite 1200

Toronto, ON M4R 1K8

Tel: 416-488-8772

Toll-free: 1-800-616-8816

E-mail: info@alzheimer.ca

Website: www.alzheimer.ca

What you'll find here:

- information on adult day programs, seminars, support groups
- The Safely Home program information: www.safelyhome.ca

Arthritis Society, The

393 University Avenue, Suite 1700

Toronto, ON M5G 1E6

Tel: 416-979-7228

E-mail: info@arthritis.ca

Website: www.arthritis.ca

Canada Mortgage and Housing Corporation

700 Montreal Road
Ottawa, ON K1A 0P7
Tel: 613-748-2000
Call Centre: 1-800-668-2642
TTY: 613-748-2447
E-mail: chic@cmhc-schl.gc.ca
Website: www.cmhc-schl.gc.ca

What you'll find here:

- information and forms on the Home Adaptation for Seniors Independence (HASI) and the Residential Rehabilitation Assistance Program (RRAP)
- "Step Through the Life-Cycle of Your Home" section, with information on programs to help seniors stay independent and in their homes, such as the self-assessment tool guide for home adaptations, tips for being at home with Alzheimer's disease, checklists and picture examples of home adaptations
- answers to frequently asked questions

Canada Safety Council

1020 Thomas Spratt Place
Ottawa, ON K1G 5L5
Tel: 613-739-1535
Website: www.safety-council.org/info/info.htm

What you'll find here:

- safety tips for seniors, driving tips, information on 55 Alive refresher courses, home adaptation, fall prevention

Canadian Association of the Deaf

251 Bank Street, Suite 203
Ottawa, ON K2P 1X3

Tel: 613-565-2882
TTY: 613-565-8882
E-mail: info@cad.ca
Website: www.cad.ca

Canadian Automobile Association: Helping Aging Drivers

Website: www.caa.ca/ainesauvolant

What you'll find here:

- tips, facts, program details, information to help you refine your skills
- regional office contact information

Canadian Cancer Society

10 Alcorn Avenue, Suite 200
Toronto, ON M4V 3B1
Tel: 416-961-7223
Toll-free: 1-888-939-3333
E-mail: ccs@cancer.ca
Website: www.cancer.ca

Canadian Caregiver Coalition

110 Argyle Avenue
Ottawa, ON K2P 1B4
Tel: 613-233-5694 ext. 2230
Toll-free: 1-888-866-2273
E-mail: info@ccc-ccan.ca
Website: www.ccc-ccan.ca

What you'll find here:

- not-for-profit organization that works to make government and the public understand the importance of caregivers in Canada

• lists of community support organizations and caregiving associations

Canadian Continence Foundation, The

P.O. Box 417
Peterborough, ON K9J 6Z3
Tel: 705-750-4600
E-mail: help@canadiancontinence.ca
Website: www.continence-fdn.ca

Canadian Hospice Palliative Care Association

Annex B, St. Vincent Hospital
60 Cambridge Street North
Ottawa, ON K1R 7A5
Tel: 613-241-3663
Toll-free: 1-800-668-2785
Info Line: 1-877-203-4636
E-mail: info@chpca.net
Website: www.chpca.net

What you'll find here:

• informal caregiver information and resources
• Canadian directory of services by city
• directory of services by province and illness
• links to palliative care associations by province

Canadian Mental Health Association

Phenix Professional Building
595 Montreal Road, Suite 303
Ottawa, ON K1K 42L
Tel: 613-745-7750
E-mail: info@cmha.ca
Website: www.cmha.ca

What you'll find here:
- support and information on aging and mental health
- information on how to cope with stress
- tips on how to find psychiatrists, psychologists, self-help groups, community services
- provincial offices locator

Canadian National Institute for the Blind (CNIB)

1929 Bayview Avenue
Toronto, ON M4G 3E8
Toll-free: 1-800-563-2642
E-mail: info@cnib.ca
Website: www.cnib.ca

Canadian Red Cross

170 Metcalfe Street, Suite 300
Ottawa, ON K2P 2P2
Tel: 613-740-1900
E-mail: feedback@redcross.ca
Website: www.redcross.ca
What you'll find here:
- links to regional contacts, home-care services, and information about borrowing assistive devices and home health care equipment

Care Guide Source for Seniors, The

20 Rivermede Road, Suite 202
Vaughan, ON L4K 3N3
Tel: 416-287-2273
Toll-free: 1-800-311-2273
Website: www.thecareguide.com

What you'll find here:

- resource centre for housing options, searchable by province (Alberta, British Columbia, Ontario)
- searchable database for independent supportive living, assisted living, long-term care residences, caregiver information and other senior-related topics

Carp

27 Queen St. East, Suite 702
Toronto, ON M5C 2M6
Tel: 416-363-8748
Toll-free: 1-800-363-9736
E-mail: carp@carp.ca
Website: www.carp.ca

What you'll find here:

- senior information and articles about topics such as advocacy, benefits and community events

Family Caregiver Newsmagazine, The

c/o Caregiver Omnimedia
2130 King Road
P.O. Box 1060
King City, ON L7B 1B1
Toll-free: 1-800-209-4810 ext. 27
Website: www.thefamilycaregiver.com

50Plus

Website: www.50plus.com

What you'll find here:

- general senior site with information on travel, health, activities, relationships and lifestyles

Financial Consumer Agency of Canada

427 Laurier Avenue West, 6th Floor

Ottawa ON K1R 1B9

Tel: 1-866-461-3222 (English)

Tel: 1-866-461-2232 (French)

Tel: 613-996-5454 (Ottawa or outside Canada)

TTY: 1-866-914-6097

TTY: 613-947-7771 (Ottawa or outside Canada)

Website: www.fcac.gc.ca

What you'll find here:

- information about banking and insurance, accounts, debit cards, standard fees; interactive tools such as cost of banking guide, tip sheets on subjects such as shopping around for a low-cost bank account, and how to protect yourself financially
- consumer information, frequently asked questions

Heart and Stroke Foundation of Canada

222 Queen Street, Suite 1402

Ottawa, ON K1P 5V9

Tel: 613-569-4361

Website: www.heartandstroke.com

March of Dimes Canada

Ontario March of Dimes

10 Overlea Boulevard

Toronto, ON M4H 1A4

Tel: 416-625-3463

Toll-free: 1-800-263-3463

E-mail: info@marchofdimes.ca

Website: www.marchofdimes.ca

What you'll find here:
- programs and services for caregivers

Osteoporosis Canada

1090 Don Mills Road, Suite 301
Toronto, ON M3C 3R6
Tel: 416-696-2663
Toll-free: 1-800-463-6842 (English)
Toll-free: 1-800-977-1778 (French)
E-mail: info@osteoporosis.ca
Website: www.osteoporosis.ca

Parkinson Society of Canada

4211 Yonge Street, Suite 316
Toronto, ON M2P 2A9
Tel: 416-227-9700
Toll-free: 1-800-565-3000
E-mail: general.info@parkinson.ca
Website: www.parkinson.ca

PhoneBusters

Box 686
North Bay, ON P1B 8J8
Toll-free: 1-888-495-8501
E-mail: info@phonebusters.com
Website: www.phonebusters.com

Salvation Army, The

2 Overlea Boulevard
Toronto, ON M4H 1P4
Tel: 416-425-2111
Website: www.salvationarmy.ca

Victorian Order of Nurses

110 Argyle Avenue

Ottawa, ON K2P 1B4

Tel: 613-233-5694

Toll-free: 1-888-866-2273

E-mail: national@von.ca

Website: www.von.ca

Caregiver web portal: www.caregiver-connect.ca

PROVINCIAL AND TERRITORIAL RESOURCES

ALBERTA

PROVINCIAL AND MUNICIPAL GOVERNMENT RESOURCES

City of Calgary Services and Programs

P.O. Box 2100, Stn. M., Mail Code #230

Calgary, AB T2P 2M5

Tel: 311 or 403-268-2489 (outside Calgary)

TTY: 403-268-4889

Website: www.calgary.ca

What you'll find here:

- search tip: go to City Living/People Resources/Seniors
- home maintenance, senior recreation centres, senior activities and senior programs and services

City of Edmonton Communications

Community Services Department

City Hall

1 Sir Winston Churchill Square, 3rd Floor

Edmonton, AB T5J 2R7

Tel: 780-944-0462

E-mail: seniors@edmonton.ca

Website: www.edmonton.ca

What you'll find here:

- search tip: go to People Services & Programs/People Services/Seniors Services
- senior centres, housing support for seniors, services available to seniors such as house maintenance

Health Link Alberta

Tel: 403-943-5465 (Calgary Health Region)

Tel: 780-408-5465 (Capital Health Region)

Toll-free: 1-866-408-5465

These are the twenty-four-hour health care phone numbers.

Website: www.healthlinkalberta.ca

What you'll find here:

- general senior health information and guide, tips, and information on caring for aging parents, dementia, how to avoid falls, staying in your home, successful aging, nutrition
- link to Meals on Wheels

Ministry of Transportation

Driver Fitness and Monitoring

Main Floor, Twin Atria Building

4999–98th Avenue

Edmonton, AB T6B 2X3

Tel: 780-427-8230

Toll-free: 780-310-0000 (Alberta)

Website: www.transportation.alberta.ca/DriversVehicles.htm

What you'll find here:

- Reports such as "Drivers: Aging Drivers," "Medical Conditions That May Affect Safe Driving," "What Happens Once a Medical is Submitted?" and "Reporting Concerns About Driver Fitness"

Office of the Public Guardian

Toll-free: 1-877-427-4525

Website: www.seniors.gov.ab.ca/contact_us/opg/index.asp

What you'll find here:

- regional listings across the province

Programs and Services

Government of Alberta

P.O. Box 1333

Edmonton, AB T5J 2N2

Tel: 780-427-2711

Toll-free: 780-310-0000 (Alberta)

TDD/TTY Toll-free: 1-800-232-7215 (Alberta)

TDD/TTY Tel: 780-427-9999 (Edmonton)

E-mail: services@gov.ab.ca

Website: www.services.gov.ab.ca

What you'll find here:

- life events section about retiring, organizations in Alberta, senior programs and services
- senior housing programs information
- transportation tips for seniors, parking permits, guides and maps
- information on provincial assistance programs: assistive devices, wheelchair modifications, health-related benefits
- senior-specific forms, for example, the Alberta Seniors Benefit Application and Special Needs Assistance for Seniors Application
- links to federal pension sites and senior benefits and assistance
- personal directive forms and links to the Public Guardian
- links to Meals on Wheels
- *Saying Farewell: A Guide to Assist You with the Death and Dying Process* handbook

Public Trustee

Justice Alberta
Tel: 780-427-2711
Toll-free: 403-310-0000 (Alberta)
Website: www.justice.gov.ab.ca

J.E. Brownlee Building
10365–97th Street, 4th Floor
Edmonton, AB T5J 3Z8
Tel: 780-427-2744

2100 Telus Tower
411–1 Street SE
Calgary, AB T2G 4Y5
Tel: 403-297-6541

Social Services Support and Assessment

Alberta Seniors and Community Supports
P.O. Box 3100
Edmonton, AB T5J 4W3
Tel: 780-427-7876 (Edmonton)
Toll-free: 1-800-642-3853 (Alberta)
TDD/TTY Toll-free: 1-800-232-7215 (Alberta)
TDD/TTY Tel: 780-427-9999 (Edmonton)
E-mail: Alberta.seniors@gov.ab.ca
Website: www.seniors.gov.ab.ca
What you'll find here:
- *Seniors Programs and Services Information Guide:*
  www.seniors.gov.ab.ca/services_resources/programs_services
- Links to housing options:
  www.seniors.gov.ab.ca/housing/seniors_housing/

Alberta Caregivers Association

Fulton Place School

10310-56 Street NW

Edmonton, AB T6A 2J2

Tel: 780-453-5800

E-mail: caregiver@albertacaregiversassociation.org

Website: www.albertacaregiversassociation.org

What you'll find here:

- general caregiver information, programs to assist the caregiver and the family, links to federal and provincial websites

Alberta Funeral Service Association

5–5431 43rd Street

Red Deer, AB T4N 1C8

Tel: 1-800-803-8809 or 403-342-2460

E-mail: inquiry@afsa.ca

Website: www.afsa.ab.ca/home.html

What you'll find here:

- information guide and answers to frequently asked questions

Family Caregiver Centre–Calgary

1509 Centre Street South

Calgary, AB T2G 2E6

Tel: 403-303-6027

E-mail: family.caregivercentre@calgaryhealthregion.ca

Website: www.calgaryhealthregion.ca/programs/famcaregiver

What you'll find here:

- tips covering a wide range of caregiving topics including medication, family meetings, power of attorney, taking care of yourself
- support groups and seminars listings
- answers to frequently asked questions specific to caregiving

BRITISH COLUMBIA
PROVINCIAL AND MUNICIPAL GOVERNMENT RESOURCES

Healthlink BC

Tel: 811 or 604-215-8110
E-mail: healthlinkbc@hlsbc.ca
Website: www.healthlinkbc.ca

BC Nurse Line

Tel: 604-215-4700 (Greater Vancouver)
Toll-free: 1-866-215-4700 (British Columbia)
TTY: 1-866-889-4700
These are the twenty-four-hour health care phone numbers.

Ministry of Healthy Living and Sport

Seniors Division
P.O. Box 9490, Stn Prov Govt
Victoria, BC V8W 9N7
Toll-free: 1-800-663-7867 (British Columbia)
Tel: 604-660-2421 (outside British Columbia)
TDD Toll-free: 1-800-661-8773
Website: www.hls.gov.bc.ca/seniors
What you'll find here:

- *BC Seniors' Guide, 8th Edition;* call with questions and to receive a copy of the booklet

Health and Seniors Information Line

Tel: 250-952-1912 (Victoria)

Toll-free: 1-800-465-4911

These are the twenty-four-hour health care phone numbers.

Ministry of Health

1515 Blanshard Street

Victoria, BC V8W 3C8

Tel: 250-952-1742 (Victoria)

Toll-free: 1-800-465-4911 (British Columbia)

E-mail: enquirybc@gov.bc.ca

Website: www.health.gov.bc.ca/seniors/

What you'll find here:

- information on medication use, fall prevention, healthy eating and healthy aging, caregiver advice, home and community care

Office of the Assisted Living Registrar

Ministry of Health

300–1275 West 6th Avenue

Vancouver, BC V6H 1A6

Tel: 605-714-3378

Toll-free: 1-866-714-3378

E-mail: info@alregistrar.bc.ca

Website: www.health.gov.bc.ca/assisted

Public Guardian and Trustee of British Columbia

700–808 West Hastings Street

Vancouver, BC V6C 3L3

Tel: 604-660-4444

or phone Service BC and ask to be transferred

Tel: 604-660-2421 (Vancouver)

Tel: 250-387-6121 (Victoria)

Toll-free: 1-800-663-7867 (British Columbia)

Fax: 604-660-0374

E-mail: mail@trustee.bc.ca

Website: www.trustee.bc.ca

Estate and Personal Trust Services

Fax: 604-660-4444

E-mail: estate@trustee.bc.ca

Social Services Support and Assessment

Ministry of Health Services

Community Care Services

Website: www.healthservices.gov.bc.ca/hcc/

What you'll find here:

- regional health authority links and contact information, which can also be found in the government pages of your phone book
- link to the Office of the Assisted Living Registrar, which has a guide to care information, lists and links

NON-GOVERNMENTAL BRITISH COLUMBIA RESOURCES

BC Housing

Suite 1701–4555 Kingsway

Burnaby, BC V5H 4V8

Tel: 604-433-2218 (Lower Mainland)

Toll-free: 1-800-257-7756

E-mail: applicantinquiries@bchousing.org

Website: www.bchousing.org/programs

Caregivers Association of BC

7731 Yukon Street
Vancouver, BC V5X 2Y4
Tel: 604-734-4812
E-mail: info@caregiver.bc.ca
Website: www.caregiverbc.ca
What you'll find here:

- links to programs across the province, tips for caregivers, and an online support group

Family Caregivers Network Society

526 Michigan Street
Victoria, BC V8V 1S2
Tel: 250-384-0408
E-mail: fcns@telus.net
Website: www.fcns-caregiving.org
What you'll find here:

- articles, local resources such as grocery delivery by phone and equipment loans, resource guide for the caregiver, resources within the province, support groups, contact numbers for long-distance caregivers

Funeral Association of British Columbia

2187 Oak Bay Avenue, Suite 211
Victoria, BC V8R 1G1
Tel: 250-592-3213
Toll-free: 1-800-665-3899
E-mail: info@bcfunerals.com
Website: www.bcfunerals.com
What you'll find here:

- information on funeral planning, estate planning, what to do when death occurs and procedures for a home death

MANITOBA

PROVINCIAL AND MUNICIPAL GOVERNMENT RESOURCES

Age Friendly Manitoba

Government of Manitoba

Tel: 204-945-3744

Toll-free: 1-866-626-4862

TTY: 204-945-4796

E-mail: mgi@gov.mb.ca

Website: www.gov.mb.ca/agefriendly

What you'll find here:

- home maintenance assistance information, community resources, information on senior centres and organizations, health services, community living, safety and security
- publications: *Senior Access Resource Manual, A Legal Information Guide for Seniors, Questions to Ask Your Doctor and Pharmacists, Older and Wiser Driver, A Guide For The Caregiver, Manitoba Seniors Guide*:
  www.gov.mb.ca/agefriendly/pdf/seniors_guide.pdf
- database of services provided by multipurpose senior centres and senior resource councils, searchable by community
- government contacts

Health Links

Tel: 204-788-8200 (Winnipeg)

Toll-free: 1-888-315-9257

These are the twenty-four-hour health care phone numbers.

Manitoba Home Care Program

Website: www.gov.mb.ca/health/homecare/

What you'll find here:
- Manitoba Home Care Program guide, information on assessments, case planning and coordination, services, personal care home placement, roles and responsibilities, home-care forms, answers to frequently asked questions

Manitoba Housing Authority

Central Office and Winnipeg Application Intake
Application Services
Main Floor–185 Smith Street
Winnipeg, MB R3C 3G4
Tel: 204-945-4663
Toll-free: 1-800-661-4663
Website: www.gov.mb.ca/fs/housing/mha.html

Minister of Health

Legislative Building
Room 302
Winnipeg, MB R3C 0V8
Tel: 204-945-3744
Toll Free: 1-866-626-4862
E-mail: minhlt@leg.gov.mb.ca
Website: www.gov.mb.ca/health

What you'll find here:
- InfoHealth guide, healthy living tips, fact sheets

Public Trustee of Manitoba

Public Trustee
Suite 500–155 Carlton Street
Winnipeg, MB R3C 5R9
Tel: 204-945-2700
E-mail: publictrustee@gov.mb.ca
Website: www.gov.mb.ca/publictrustee/

Social Services Support and Assessment

Seniors and Healthy Aging Secretariat

822–155 Carlton Street

Winnipeg, MB R3C 3H8

Tel: 204-945-6565 (Winnipeg)

Toll-free: 1-800-665-6565 (Manitoba)

Fax: 204-948-2514

E-mail: seniors@gov.mb.ca

Website: www.gov.mb.ca/shas

What you'll find here:

- call to receive a booklet copy of the *Manitoba Seniors Guide*: www.gov.mb.ca/agefriendly/pdf/seniors_guide.pdf
- regional health authority contact information: www.gov.mb.ca/health/rha/contact.html

NON-GOVERNMENTAL MANITOBA RESOURCES

Manitoba Funeral Service Association

P.O. Box 243

Winnipeg, MB R3C 2G9

Tel: 204-947-0927

Website: www.mfsa.mb.ca/index.php

NEW BRUNSWICK

PROVINCIAL AND MUNICIPAL GOVERNMENT RESOURCES

New Brunswick Health

HSBC Place

P.O. Box 5100

Fredericton, NB E3B 5G8

Tel: 506-457-4800

E-mail: hw_sme@gnb.ca

Website: www.gnb.ca/0051

What you'll find here:

- a senior-specific information section with program information, forms and caregiving tips

Office of the Public Trustee

P.O. Box 400

Fredericton, NB E3B 4Z9

Tel: 506-444-3688

Toll-free: 1-888-336-8383

E-mail: public.trustee@gnb.ca

Website: www.gnb.ca/0062/PT-CP/index-e.asp

Service New Brunswick

Westmoreland Place

82 Westmoreland Street

Fredericton, NB E3B 3L3

Tel: 506-444-2897

Toll-free: 1-888-762-8600

Website: www.gnb.ca

What you'll find here:

- search tip: go to Individuals and Families/Seniors
- a caregiving booklet, and a senior guide to services and programs; information on senior care such as housing options, legal concerns, recognizing elder abuse, financial aid, medical programs

Social Services Support and Assessment

Department of Social Development

Sartain MacDonald Building

P.O. Box 6000

Fredericton, NB E3B 5H1

Tel: 506-453-2001

Website: www.gnb.ca/0017/Seniors/index-e.asp

What you'll find here:

- contact list by region for family and community services offices
- link to supportive housing: www.gnb.ca/0017/Housing/index-e.asp

TeleCare

Toll-free: 1-800-244-8353

This is the twenty-four-hour health care phone number.

NEWFOUNDLAND AND LABRADOR

PROVINCIAL AND MUNICIPAL GOVERNMENT RESOURCES

City of St. John's

City Hall

10 New Gower Street

P.O. Box 908

St. John's, NL A1C 5M2

Tel: 311 or 709-754-2489

Website: www.stjohns.ca/cityservices/seniors/index.jsp

What you'll find here:

- Seniors Resource Centre, senior programs and recreation such as community programs, special events and senior discount application form

Communications Branch

General Inquiries

10th Floor, East Block

Confederation Building
St. John's, NL A1B 4J6
Tel: 709-729-2300 (call collect)

What you'll find here:

- senior resource links, pension information and low-income senior benefit program information
- Services Directory: www.gov.nl.ca/services

HealthLine

Tel: 1-888-709-2929
TTY: 1-888-709-3555

These are the twenty-four-hour health care phone numbers.

Seniors Resource Centre Association of Newfoundland and Labrador

280 Torbay Road, Suite W100
St. John's, NL A1A 3W8
Tel: 709-737-2333
Toll-free: 1-800-563-5599 (Newfoundland and Labrador)
E-mail: info@seniorsresource.ca
Website: www.seniorsresource.ca

What you'll find here:

- senior programs, support groups, publications, provincial programs
- senior guide to services and programs
- "Caregivers Out of Isolation" has a caregiver hotline (1-800-571-2273), advice for caregivers, resources and special events: www.seniorsresource.ca/caregivers/

Social Services Support and Assessment

Department of Health and Community Services
1st Floor, West Block
Confederation Building

P.O. Box 8700

St. John's, NL A1B 4J6

Tel: 709-729-4984

E-mail: healthinfo@gov.nl.ca

Website: www.health.gov.nl.ca/health

What you'll find here:

- services delivered by the regional Health and Community Services/Integrated Health Care Boards

NORTHWEST TERRITORIES
TERRITORIAL AND MUNICIPAL GOVERNMENT RESOURCES

Government of the Northwest Territories

Centre Square Tower, 8th Floor

5022–49th Street

P.O. Box 1320

Yellowknife, NT X1A 2L9

Tel: 867-873-7500

Website: www.hlthss.gov.nt.ca/seniors

What you'll find here:

- Social Services Support and Assessment section through the Department of Health and Social Services; contact the Seniors Information Line
- information on senior benefits, housing programs, health benefits and application forms; links to federal and provincial programs, senior clubs and organizations
- *Seniors' Information Handbook*: www.hlthss.gov.nt.ca/pdf/reports/seniors/2008/english/seniors_information_handbook_2008.pdf

Office of the Public Trustee

P.O. Box 1320

Yellowknife, NT X1A 2L9

Tel: 867-873-7464

Website: www.justice.gov.nt.ca/PublicTrustee/index.shtml

Tele-Care Health Line

Tel: 1-888-255-1010

TTY: 1-888-255-8211

These are the twenty-four-hour health care phone numbers.

NON-GOVERNMENTAL NORTHWEST TERRITORIES RESOURCES

NWT Senior's Society

4916–46th Street, Suite 102

Yellowknife, NT X1A 1L2

Tel: 867-920-7444

Toll-free: 1-800-661-0878

E-mail: seniors@yk.com

Website: www.nwtseniorssociety.ca

What you'll find here:

• information and resources, links

NOVA SCOTIA

PROVINCIAL AND MUNICIPAL GOVERNMENT RESOURCES

Department of Seniors, The

Dennis Building, 4th Floor

1740 Granville Street

P.O. Box 2065

Halifax, NS B3J 2Z1

Tel: 902-424-0065 (metro area)

Toll-free: 1-800-670-0065

E-mail: scs@gov.ns.ca

Website: www.gov.ns.ca/scs

What you'll find here:

- listing of government programs; information on services for seniors, housing and health
- *Programs for Seniors 2008*: www.gov.ns.ca/scs/programs.asp

Nova Scotia Public Trustee

Public Trustee Office

405–5670 Spring Garden Road

P.O. Box 685

Halifax, NS B3J 2T3

Tel: 902-424-7760

Website: www.gov.ns.ca/just/public_trustee.asp

Social Services Support and Assessment

Department of Health

Continuing Care Services

1690 Hollis Street

Halifax, NS B3J 2R8

Toll-free: 1-800-225-7225 (Nova Scotia)

Tel: 902-424-4288 (outside Nova Scotia)

Website: www.gov.ns.ca/health/ccs/

What you'll find here:

- list of contacts by region
- Community Services, and regional office contact information for the Housing Authority: www.gov.ns.ca/coms/housing/rental/SeniorsRentalHousing.html

Caregivers Nova Scotia

Tower 1, Suite 105

7001 Mumford Road

Halifax, NS B3L 4N9

Tel: 902-421-7390

Toll-free: 1-877-488-7390 (Nova Scotia)

Website: www.caregiversns.org

What you'll find here:

- support groups, events, caregiver online forum and a caregiver planning guide

NUNAVUT
TERRITORIAL AND MUNICIPAL GOVERNMENT RESOURCES

Department of Justice

Legal and Constitutional Division

Government of Nunavut

P.O. Box 1000, Station 540

Iqaluit, NU X0A 0H0

Tel: 867-975-6320

Fax: 867-975-6349

E-mail: justice.legal@gov.nu.ca

Website: www.justice.gov.nu.ca/english/legalcons.html

Government of Nunavut

Toll-free: 1-888-252-9869

Social Services Support and Assessment

Department of Health and Social Services

Government of Nunavut

P.O. Box 1000, Station 1000

Iqaluit, NU X0A 0H0

Tel: 867-975-5700

Website: www.gov.nu.ca/health

ONTARIO

PROVINCIAL AND MUNICIPAL GOVERNMENT RESOURCES

City of Ottawa

Services for Seniors

110 Laurier Avenue West

Ottawa, ON K1P 1J1

Tel: 311 or 613-580-2400

Toll-free: 1-866-261-9799

TTY: 613-580-2401

Website: www.ottawa.ca/residents/seniors

What you'll find here:

• listing of city services, senior centres, safety tips, transportation and mobility options, housing information

City of Toronto

Seniors Portal

Tel: 416-338-0338

TTY: 416-338-0TTY (0889)

Fax: 416-338-0685

E-mail: accesstoronto@toronto.ca

Website: www.toronto.ca/seniors

What you'll find here:
- information on accommodation, getting around, health, lifelong learning, and safety, plus publications and answers to frequently asked questions

Long-Term Care Action Line

Tel: 1-866-434-0144

TTY: 1-800-387-5559

Ministry of Health and Long-Term Care

Service Ontario INFOline

M-1B114, Macdonald Block

900 Bay Street

Toronto, ON M7A 1N3

Toll-free: 1-866-532-3161

Website: www.health.gov.on.ca

What you'll find here:
- general health care information; senior care section with information on housing and care, homemaking, finding a CCAC centre, long-term-care home reports, tips for providers, resources and links
- link to supportive housing: www.health.gov.on.ca/english/public/program/ltc/13_housing.html

Ministry of Transportation

Queen's Park/Minister's Office

77 Wellesley Street West

Ferguson Block, 3rd Floor

Toronto, ON M7A 1Z8

Tel: 416-327-9200

Website: www.mto.gov.on.ca

What you'll find here:
- publications such as *How's Your Driving? Safe Driving for Seniors*: www.mto.gov.on.ca/english/pubs/seniorguide/index.shtml

Office of the Public Guardian and Trustee Ontario

Ministry of the Attorney General

McMurtry-Scott Building

720 Bay Street, 11th Floor

Toronto, ON M5G 2K1

Tel: 416-326-2220

Toll-free: 1-800-518-7901

TTY: 416-326-4012

Website: www.attorneygeneral.jus.gov.on.ca/english/family/pgt/

What you'll find here:
- listing of city services, information on senior centres, transportation and mobility options, housing, and safety tips

Ontario Seniors' Secretariat

777 Bay Street, Suite 601C

Toronto, ON M7A 2J4

Toll-free: 1-888-910-1999

TTY: 1-800-387-5559

Website: www.ontarioseniors.ca

What you'll find here:
- programs and services, information and resources, listings of senior organizations and senior centres, seminars on fall safety and driving
- *A Guide to Programs and Services for Seniors in Ontario*: www.culture.gov.on.ca/seniors/english/programs/seniorsguide

Social Services Support and Assessment

Community Care Access Centre (CCAC)

Contact your regional office, which can also be found in the government pages of your phone book

Website: www.ccac-ont.ca

What you'll find here:

- social services support and assessment
- programs and services information

Telehealth Ontario

Toll-free: 1-866-797-0000

TTY: 1-866-797-0007

These are the twenty-four-hour health care phone numbers.

Website: www.health.gov.on.ca

NON-GOVERNMENTAL ONTARIO RESOURCES

Board of Funeral Services

777 Bay Street, Suite 2810

Box 117

Toronto, ON M5G 2C8

Tel: 416-979-5450

Toll-free: 1-800-387-4458

E-mail: info@funeralboard.com

Website: www.funeralboard.com

Ontario Long-Term Care Association (OLTCA)

345 Renfrew Drive, 3rd Floor

Markham, ON L3R 9S9

Tel: 905-470-8995

Website: www.oltca.com

What you'll find here:

- an association of long term care providers—private, not-for-profit, charitable and municipal—in Ontario
- listing of associated members, general information and resources

Ontario Retirement Communities Association

2155 Leanne Boulevard, Suite 218

Mississauga, ON L5K 2K8

Tel: 905-403-0500

Toll-free: 1-800-361-7254

Website: www.orca-homes.com

What you'll find here:

- a voluntary non-profit organization that sets professional operating standards, and inspects and accredits retirement residences in Ontario
- listing of members, tips on how to choose a home, information on housing standards

Ontario Seniors' Info

Website: www.seniorsinfo.ca

What you'll find here:

- a collaborative online portal for information for seniors in Ontario
- e-forms, information on end of life, links to housing options, in-home care, caregiving associations

PRINCE EDWARD ISLAND

PROVINCIAL AND MUNICIPAL GOVERNMENT RESOURCES

Department of Transportation and Public Works

Government of Prince Edward Island

3rd Floor, Jones Building

11 Kent Street

P.O. Box 2000

Charlottetown, PEI C1A 7N8

Tel: 902-368-5228

What you'll find here:

- "Drive Safely as You Age" pamphlet:
  www.gov.pe.ca/tpwpei/index.php3?number=1001823&lang=E

Office of the Public Guardian and Public Trustee

Shaw Building

95–105 Rochford Street

Charlottetown, PEI C1A 7N8

Tel: 902-368-4561 (Office of the Deputy Public Trustee)

Tel: 902-368-6506 (Office of the Public Guardian)

Website: www.gov.pe.ca/infopei/index.php3?number=43209&lang=E

Prince Edward Island Seniors' Secretariat

Department of Social Services and Seniors

2nd Floor, Jones Building

11 Kent Street

P.O. Box 2000

Charlottetown, PEI C1A 7N8

Tel: 902-569-0588 (Charlottetown)

Toll-free: 1-866-770-0588

E-mail: seniors@gov.pe.ca

Website: www.gov.pe.ca/seniors

What you'll find here:

- an extensive senior information site that offers a caregiver information handbook, and information on finances, housing options, services for seniors such as day programs, meal services, home adaptations, and tax benefits
- *Prince Edward Island Seniors' Guide*:

  www.gov.pe.ca/infopei/index.php3?number=1020792&lang=E

Social Services Support and Assessment

Department of Health

Government of Prince Edward Island

16 Garfield Street, 1st Floor

P.O. Box 2000

Charlottetown, PEI C1A 7N8

Tel: 902-368-6130

Website: www.gov.pe.ca/health

What you'll find here:

- contacts for home-care offices by region
- database searchable by community programs and services

QUEBEC

PROVINCIAL AND MUNICIPAL GOVERNMENT RESOURCES

Curateur public Québec

(Public Trustee)

600, boulevard René-Lévesque Ouest, 12e étage

Montréal, QC H3B 4W9

Tel: 514-873-4074

Toll-free: 1-800-363-9020

E-mail: information@curateur.gouv.qc.ca

Website: www.curateur.gouv.qc.ca

Info-Santé

Tel: 811

This is the twenty-four-hour health care phone number.

Justice Québec

Édifice Louis-Philippe-Pigeon

1200, route de l'Église, 6e étage

Québec, QC G1V 4M1

Tel: 418-643-5140

Toll-free: 1-866-536-5140

E-mail: informations@justice.gouv.qc.ca

Website: www.justice.gouv.qc.ca

What you'll find here:

• information on wills and the *What to Do in the Event of Death* guide:

www.deces.info.gouv.qc.ca/en/publications/deces_en.pdf

Services Québec

Government of Québec

Tel: 418-644-4545 (Québec City)

Tel: 514-644-4545 (Montréal)

Toll-free: 1-877-644-4545 (Québec)

Website: www.55ans.info.gouv.qc.ca

What you'll find here:

• general information on housing options, health care, driving, assistive devices

Social Services Support and Assessment

Ministère de la Santé et des Services Sociaux Québec

(Health and Social Services Québec)

Government of Québec

Tel: 418-644-4545 (Québec City)

Tel: 514-644-4545 (Montréal)

Toll-free: 1-877-644-4545 (Québec)

TTY: 514-873-4626 (Montréal)

TTY Toll-free: 1-800-361-9596 (Québec)

Website: www.msss.gouv.qc.ca/en/sujets/groupes/seniors.php

What you'll find here:

- Registre des Résidences pour Personnes Âgées (The Register of Residences for Seniors); reports on long-term care facilities in the province and a map locator of homes: http://wpp01.msss.gouv.qc.ca/appl/K10/K10accueil.asp

Société d'habitation Québec

(Affordable Housing Québec–Social and Community Component)

Government of Québec

Website:www.habitation.gouv.qc.ca/en/programmes/volet_social.html

SASKATCHEWAN

PROVINCIAL AND MUNICIPAL GOVERNMENT RESOURCES

HealthLine

Tel: 1-877-800-0002

TTY: 1-888-425-4444

These are the twenty-four-hour health care phone numbers.

Health Saskatchewan

Government of Saskatchewan

Website: www.health.gov.sk.ca/seniors

What you'll find here:

- senior health information, senior chat column, health benefits, senior programs and services guide

Public Guardian and Trustee

Justice and Attorney General Saskatchewan

Government of Saskatchewan

100–1871 Smith Street

Regina, SK S4P 4W4

Tel: 306-787-5424

Toll-free: 1-877-787-5424

E-mail: pgt@gov.sk.ca

Website: www.justice.gov.sk.ca/pgt

Social Services Saskatchewan

Government of Saskatchewan

Website: www.socialservices.gov.sk.ca/seniors

What you'll find here:

- information about programs and services for seniors
- information about housing options
- links to affordable housing rentals and Saskatchewan Assisted Living Services (SALS)
- regional office contact information, which can be found in the government pages of your phone book

Social Services Support and Assessment

Health Saskatchewan

Community Care Branch

Government of Saskatchewan

3475 Albert Street, 1st Floor

Regina, SK S4S 6X6

Tel: 306-787-7239

Website: www.health.gov.sk.ca/continuing-care

NON-GOVERNMENTAL SASKATCHEWAN RESOURCES

Saskatoon Caregiver Information Centre

Saskatoon Council on Aging

Community Service Village

#301–506 25th Street East

Saskatoon, SK S7K 4A7

Tel: 306-652-4411

E-mail: caregiver@sasktel.net

Website: www.caregive.sasktelwebsite.net

What you'll find here:

• general caregiver information

• caregiver guide with tips and caregiver websites, answers to frequently asked questions, directory of services and social activities for seniors

YUKON

TERRITORIAL AND MUNICIPAL GOVERNMENT RESOURCES

HealthLine

Tel: 811

This is the twenty-four-hour health care phone number.

Office of the Public Guardian and Trustee

Mailing address:

Department of Justice

Government of Yukon

P.O. Box 2703 (J-2B)

Whitehorse, YT Y1A 2C6

Location:

Andrew A. Philipsen Law Centre

3rd Floor

2130–2nd Avenue

Whitehorse, YT Y1A 2C6

Tel: 867-667-5366

Toll-free: 1-800-661-0408 ext. 5366 (Yukon)

E-mail: publicguardianandtrustee@gov.yk.ca

Website: www.publicguardianandtrustee.gov.yk.ca

Programs and Services for Seniors

Government of Yukon

Tel: 867-667-5811

Toll-free: 1-800-661-0408 (outside Whitehorse)

Website: www.gov.yk.ca/services/people_seniors.html

What you'll find here:

- list of community health centres, day programs, home care, respite care, crime prevention for seniors, housing programs like yard maintenance, the Pharmacare and Extended Benefits program and extended health care benefits

Social Services Support and Assessment

Health and Social Services

Government of Yukon

P.O. Box 2703

Whitehorse, YT Y1A 2C6

Tel: 867-667-3673

Toll-free: 1-800-661-0408 ext. 3673 (Yukon)

E-mail: hss@gov.yk.ca

Website: www.hss.gov.yk.ca/seniors

What you'll find here:

- information about Yukon Home Care Program

- contact the Admissions/Assessments Coordinator (867-667-8961) for information on eligibility

The authors have made every attempt to provide the correct contact information and are not responsible for information on these websites.

ENDNOTES

1. Source: Statistics Canada, Kelly Cranswick, *General Social Survey, Cycle 16: Caring for an Aging Society,* Catalogue no. 89–582, 2003, 11.

2. Source: "What Is a Family/Informal Caregiver?" Health Canada, 2002. Reproduced with the permission of the Minister of Public Works and Government Services Canada, 2008.

3. Source: Philippe Le Goff, *Home Care Sector in Canada: Economic Problems,* Economic Division Catalogue no. PRB 02–29E, 2002.

4. Source: "National Profile of Family Caregivers in Canada—2002 Final Report," Health Canada, 2002. Reproduced with the permission of the Minister of Public Works and Government Services Canada, 2008.

5. Source: Statistics Canada, Grant Schellenberg and Martin Turcotte, *A Portrait of Seniors in Canada,* Catalogue no. 89–519-XWE, 2006, 12.

6. Source: Statistics Canada, Grant Schellenberg and Martin Turcotte, *A Portrait of Seniors in Canada,* Catalogue no. 89–519-XWE, 2006, 13.

7. Source: Statistics Canada, Grant Schellenberg and Martin Turcotte, *A Portrait of Seniors in Canada,* Catalogue no. 89–519-XWE, 2006, 44.

8. Source: Statistics Canada, The Daily, "A Portrait of Seniors," www.statcan.ca/Daily/English/070227/d070227b.htm (accessed April 2, 2008).

9. Source: Statistics Canada, Grant Schellenberg and Martin Turcotte, *A Portrait of Seniors in Canada,* Catalogue no. 89–519-XWE, 2006, 212.

10. Source: Statistics Canada, Grant Schellenberg and Martin Turcotte, *A Portrait of Seniors in Canada,* Catalogue no. 89–519-XWE, 2006, 50.

11. Source: "The Safe Living Guide: A Guide to Home Safety for Seniors, 3rd Edition," Public Health Agency of Canada, 2008, 4. Reproduced with the permission of the Minister of Public Works and Government Services Canada, 2008.

12. Source: "The Safe Living Guide: A Guide to Home Safety for Seniors," Public Health Agency of Canada, 2005, 8. Revised and reproduced with the permission of the Minister of Public Works and Government Services Canada, 2009.

13. Source: The Alzheimer Society of Canada, "Alzheimer's Disease: 10 Warning Signs," www.alzheimer.ca/english/disease/warningsigns .htm (accessed May 15, 2008).

14. Source: "Enhancing Safety and Security for Canadian Seniors: Setting the Stage for Action," Public Health Agency of Canada, 1999, 18. Reproduced with the permission of the Minister of Public Works and Government Services Canada, 2008.

15. Source: "Financial Abuse of Older Adults," Public Health Agency of Canada, 2005, 8. Revised and reproduced with the permission of the Minister of Public Works and Government Services Canada, 2009.

16. Source: "Financial Abuse of Older Adults," Public Health Agency of Canada, 2005, 8. Revised and reproduced with the permission of the Minister of Public Works and Government Services Canada, 2009.

Any errors or omissions, please contact the publisher.

INDEX

Activities of Daily Living. *See*
    ADL
ADL (Activities of Daily Living),
    51–53
aging
    appetite and, 37
    common conditions associated
      with, 142–47
    early signs of, 13
    increasing time needed for tasks
      with, 138
    perceptual acuity and (*See also*
      hearing difficulties; vision
      difficulties)
    physical decline with, 129–30
Alzheimer's disease, 2, 38, 68, 111,
    143, 147, 172
anxiety, aging and, 143–45
arthritis, 143
assistive devices (for walking,
    seeing, hearing, etc.), 86–88

banking
    electronic, 160–63
    seniors and, 159–60

cancer, 143
care facilities (*See also* home moving)
    checklists for, 106–7, 121–23
    safety in, 120
    selecting among, 99–101, 105–8,
      114–23
caregivers (*See also* caregiving)
    avoiding burnout among, 196–99
    children of, 56, 69–74, 112
    conflicts among, 56–67
    demographics of, 10
    doctors and, 132, 135–39, 141–42
    feelings of inadequacy in, 19
    guilt felt by, 4, 23, 57, 108–9, 116,
      123, 126, 149, 151, 184–85,
      190–91, 197–99
    hospital visits and, 149–50
    maintaining effectiveness as,
      184–85, 188–99
    needs for support of, 3–6
    numbers of, 3, 8
    professional, 5, 88–94
    resources available to (*See also*
      seniors, resources available
      to), 9, 39, 41, 91–92, 152, 159,
      166, 193–94, 209–51

selection of professional, 94–96

social impacts of, 3, 10, 21–22

spouses or partners of, 67–69,
108–11

support for, 152, 154–56

caregiving (*See also* caregivers)

differing perceived needs for,
57–58, 123

dignity as a primary goal of,
16–18, 28–29, 125, 142

economics and, 9

family sizes and, 3

financial assistance and (*See also*
finances), 33–34, 158–67

full time in the parent's own
home, 123–24

as gratitude and thanks, 74, 113,
187, 192, 201, 204–6

health impacts upon caregivers
from, 9

independence as a primary goal
of, 16–18, 28–31, 42, 45, 78,
80, 125, 142

"informal," 9, 89–90

in your own home, 108–13

living in your parent's home,
113–14

medical needs and, 21, 128–42,
173

moving parents and. *See* home
moving

pain management and, 152

planning for, 20, 206

psychological impacts on
caregivers from (*See also*
caregivers, avoiding burnout
among; caregiving, stresses
associated with), 9, 11, 15–16

recognizing the needs for, 19–21,
26, 36–37

requirements for successful,
15–20, 26–27

respectful approaches to, 13–15

rewards of, 10, 14, 17, 23, 74–75,
100, 113, 124, 185, 187, 192,
201, 204–5

social and societal effects of, 9

stages of, 20–22

stresses associated with (*See also*
caregivers, maintaining effec-
tiveness as), 9, 21–22, 57–60,
69–70, 131, 141, 184–201

terminal stages of, 22

childhood, enduring roles associated
with, 18–19, 27–28, 35, 54,
59–60, 89, 94, 109, 147

children (*See also* caregivers,
children of)

readings about aging for, 71–72

communication (with aging
parents)

importance of, 26–28, 35–37, 40,
46, 51, 54, 93–94, 100, 125, 142

potential obstacles to, 28–35

compassionate care leave (from
work), 155–56, 193–94

day programs, for seniors, 51

death of a parent, information
needed following, 180–82

dementia, 143, 147, 186–87

dependency, personal difficulties
presented by, 16–18

depression, aging and, 36, 51, 130,
143, 145–46

diabetes, 143

diet, importance of (*See also* meals),
    141
dignity (*See also* caregiving, dignity
    as a primary goal of)
    different perspectives about, 28
    personal difficulties presented by
        loss of, 16–18, 86
doctors
    appointments with, 12
    caregivers and. *See* caregivers,
        doctors and
driving (automobiles)
    alternatives to, 46–47
    cessation of, 12, 41–47, 68
Dunn, Barbara, 2–5, 8, 64, 66, 101,
    103, 114, 133, 161, 205

eating. *See* meals
employers, employees as caregivers
    and, 154, 192–94
estate planning (*See also* wills
    [legal]), 167
exercise
    for the caregiver, 195
    health and, 129, 141, 144

falling
    dangers and injuries from,
        78–80
    prevention of, 80–81, 83
family dynamics
    allowances needed for, 31–32,
        56–60, 108–15, 123, 129–30
    growth of and in, 70
    resolving conflicts due to, 61–67,
        102
family meetings, 63–67
feeding. *See* meals

finances (*See also* caregiving,
    financial)
    home selling and, 102
    management of by seniors, 53
The Financial Consumer Agency of
    Canada, 159
fire safety, 83
foot problems, 143
funerals, 178–80

gardening, 49, 126
geriatric assessments, 147–49
gerontologists, 148
    environmental, 86
government inspection reports (care
    facilities), 120
guilt. *See* caregivers, guilt felt by

health issues. *See* aging; caregiving;
    family dynamics; meals
hearing difficulties, aging and, 79,
    88, 131, 136, 143–44
heart disease, 45, 140, 143
history (personal), sharing of, 73–74
hobbies for seniors, 48
home, maintaining residence at, 12,
    78–96
home moving (*See also* care facili-
    ties; home selling)
    to an assisted living facility,
        114–15
    to condominiums or apartments,
        103–4
    to life-lease housing, 104–5
    to a long-term care home, 115–23
    psychological stresses caused by,
        98, 101, 104–5, 124–25
    reasons for, 98, 100–101

to a relative's home, 108–13

to retirement or care residences,
105–8

strategies for easing, 99, 101–3

home selling, 101–2

hospice care, 153

hospital visits, 139

emergency, 149–50, 152

housekeeping, assistance with, 41

humour, helpful roles of, 73, 88, 196

hygiene, aging parents and, 53

IADL (Instrumental Activities of
Daily Living), 51–52

incontinence, 143

independence (*See also* caregiving,
independence as a primary
goal of)

different perspectives concerning, 28–29, 42

Instrumental Activities of Daily
Living. *See* IADL

the Internet, benefits to seniors
provided by, 12–13, 48, 163

lawyers. *See* legal issues; power(s) of
attorney; wills (legal)

legal issues, caregiving and, 32–33

life expectancies, Canadian, 12

the "Living Will," Canadian alternatives to, 174

loneliness, aging and, 130, 143, 145–46

meals

as evidence of parental needs,
36–37

for the caregiver, 194

simplifying the preparation of,
38–39, 190–91

Meals on Wheels (service), 39, 191

medical notebook, utility of a,
137–38, 141

medications

driving and, 43

management of by seniors, 54,
132–35, 140–41

sleep disturbances and, 145

memories, sharing of, 73–75

memory loss, 143–44

assistance overcoming, 88

difficulties with, 54, 79

doctor's advice and, 136

effects of on medication
routines, 133–35

mobility, management of by seniors,
54

moving aging parents. *See* home
moving

music, 50, 100, 144, 196

nursing homes. *See* home moving, to
a long-term care home

organ donation, wishes concerning,
33, 174–75

osteoporosis, 143

pain management. *See* caregiving,
pain management and

palliative care, 152–55

parenting, enduring roles associated
with, 27–29, 35, 114

pharmacists, assistance from,
134–35, 138

planning for parental care. *See* caregiving, planning for
power(s) of attorney, 2, 32–33, 136,
 149, 167–76
Public Guardian and Trustee,
 166–67, 177

readings suggested re. aging, for
 children, 71–72
recreation for seniors, 48, 120
respite care support for caregivers,
 198–99
resuscitation, wishes and orders
 concerning, 33, 174
retirement, 10, 33–34, 50
routine (daily), disorientation
 following changes in, 130

Safely Home program, 147
safety (*See also* security, financial
 care facilities and), 120
 home, 37, 78–88
 road, 42–46
Scott, Linda, 2–5, 8, 14, 36, 50, 81,
 145, 160, 182, 206
security
 financial, 161, 163–68, 170–71
 of possessions, 165

seniors
 demographics of, 10, 12
 resources available to (*See also*
  caregivers, resources available
  to), 45
shopping
 assistance with, 12, 39
 groceries and, 39–40
sleeping problems, 143, 145–46
social contacts, aging parents and,
 36, 38, 47–51, 53, 129–30
special-care homes. *See* home
 moving, to a long-term care
 home
spouses. *See* caregivers, spouses or
 partners of
strokes, 143

Tear Soup (book), 180
thinking, disorientation in, 79
time management, 189–90

vision difficulties, aging and, 135, 143
volunteering, by seniors, 48

walkers, types of, 87
wills (legal), 3, 32, 176–78